FOREVER YOUTHFUL

FEEL LIKE A YOUNG PERSON FOR THE REST OF YOUR LIFE

STEVE WATSON

"Forever Youthful"

- *What is infection, where does it stem from, how dangerous can it become?*
- *Transplants, are they the final analyses of the effect of arthritis?*
- *Digestion and nutrition: two full chapters, one on each of these two important subjects.*
- *Constipation the end result of drinking too little water?*
- *Constipation: a serious condition that can have dire consequences to one's health.*
- *Healthy body cells, how important are they and how are they achieved?*
- *A healthy vascular system: the answer to a fantastic life style?*
- *Haemorrhoids, avoid the worst pain ever.*
- *Healthy children should be our ultimate mission in life.*
- *Irrigation of the colon, there are easier ways.*
- *Hollow tooth and no pain, how is that possible? Read on.*
- *Give elderly family members/friends a new lease on life.*
- *Hot/cold therapy: the easy way out?*
- *"I am very regular" not the point.*
- *We dig our grave with our teeth.*
- *A sharp memory for life*

All of the above and plenty more – 23 chapters in all.

Note

Although it is recommended that reading should start with the introduction, as each chapter is a different subject, any chapter can be read first.

This book is written in an easy-to-read conversational style, just you and I having a nice chat.

During our retirement years, we feed off memories. Memories decide the quality of our lives during that time of life, which can be extensive. *Be sure to create memories that will ensure a happy and contented old age. Old age does not start after retirement, it begins at birth. The next 70 + years will prove how good we were at securing a comfortable old age. The proof will be in the pudding. The younger we start the better, the more material will be available to work with.*

At the age I am now, I come into contact with many retired folks. I usually sit and listen rather than take part in the repartee. It almost always run along the same lines: aches and pains, blood pressure gone through the roof, pacemakers, stents, and whatever else could possibly go wrong, most caused by bad eating habits. It is as easy to adopt good as it is to adopt bad in everything, in thought, word or deed.

Then I think to myself... it could have been so different. Just a few simple changes to their lifestyle, nothing mind-blowing. Surely it would have been worth that tiny little effort; certainly no sacrifice. That is not the time in life to be caught off-guard. Let's just put it down to not knowing.

Here is an opportunity to become more enlightened. Should you have youth on your side, make the effort not to fall into that trap. It is never too late! You may have eaten yourself sick; now eat yourself well again. There may still be enough left to improve. As long as there is life left to work with, it is not too late!!!

Read on and learn how to save yourself from a miserable old age.

I cannot substantiate my theory, apart from conviction from personal experience and advice that turned out to be successful to others, that these toxins (which are more like poison by now) can be responsible for causing all sorts of problems, for instance forming crystals that lead to many different maladies that originate from inside the body. Arthritis comes to mind, which is just one of many.

Table of Contents

Preface

Artists are born and not made. These are my convictions, which often leave me with a feeling of being unfulfilled. Yes, I do have a passion for the arts, any form of art. I discovered that writing, something I enjoy enormously, is also considered to be a form of art. Inspired by reading, one of my great loves, writing has provided me with lots of joy ever since. Unlike most art forms, when they have been completed there is no going back. That is an aspect of writing I appreciate and enjoy very much. I can rewrite and change at will. It is great to be part of the world of art.

The following is my way of bringing to the world a simple and easy way of recognizing and appreciating the great gift of good health and the importance of looking after not only the body, but the entire existence, and enjoying the benefits of a life that guarantees so much more to daily living.

When opening a book, magazine, or any related writing on the subject, "health" is as a matter of course littered with scientific or outlandish words the average person has no idea the meaning of. To even further confuse the average reader and income earner, the food or ingredients to prepare these equally outlandish dishes are usually very expensive and only obtainable from upmarket stores.

When I put myself into the shoes of these individuals to whom and to what purpose the writing is aimed, without exception it seems to be a case of preaching to the converted and those who can afford it.

That inspired me to write a book that will not only prove to the average person it is possible to enjoy a high standard of good health with what is available at prices they can afford, but which includes guidelines to achieve a positive, prosperous, and healthy mindset as well.

Life is precious... that nobody will dispute. Life can also be beautiful, it can be good, it can be great. It is within everyone's ability to achieve this wonderful state of being. It is not only reserved for the rich, intellectual, or academic elite. All that is required is for someone to teach the individual how all that can be achieved. It starts with self-belief and the confidence of the individual in his/her ability to make it a reality.

You will discover it is not at all difficult to achieve that level of confidence in a very short period of time. The objective is to snare the attention of the average and disadvantaged individual, who has probably never spared a thought that he/she could enjoy a better life, and so bring about a change towards a more interesting and successful existence.

While reading how to go about achieving your goals may at times seem a bit in the extreme, looking at it on a scale from one to ten makes a little more sense. If you are serious about finding the best that life can offer and are not afraid to commit yourself to the task of finding the treasures that will make your dreams come true, you will without a doubt look forward to the challenge of tackling a ten.

For the less ambitious who would still like to have a go at improving their lifestyle, the scale will still have some merit and they can commit themselves to whatever level suits them. Even the not so young can also achieve some benefit. Everybody wins.

There are many categories, and it is not necessary to commit to all of them. Even if it is merely the idea of a better diet that is appealing, they will be a whole lot better off than they are now. Any person of any age and any level of fitness whose conscience has been stirred, will find some way of benefitting from the knowledge they have gained. All that is required is a commitment, and hopefully, we will be able to motivate them to accept a longer-term challenge, however big or small.

***THIS BOOK IS FOR ALL AGES EVERY BODY CAN OR WILL BENEFIT FROM IT**, more so our average younger brothers and sisters, who have much more to gain from what they will learn. Many budding geniuses may just become aware of the fact that they also may have an opportunity to achieve success in spite of their present state of existence, and develop themselves to their full all-round potential. The younger they are, the more they have to gain. They have time on their side. Let us find those candidates as early as possible during their lifetime.*

You will not find any mind-blowing formulae or way-out ideas that promise overnight miracles. The program is based on simple common sense, or perhaps "common sense that is not so common." Common sense needs to be exposed and stirred up sometimes, and even that can be achieved with down-to-earth methods; nothing earth-shattering.

Even when an objective is staring them in the face, some people still can't see the wood for the trees until they are shown how. Some time or other all of us have some nagging thought with potential in the back of our minds, constantly begging for attention which it does not receive until something stirs our imagination. Once we have gained just a modicum of confidence and have learned to act upon it, which is the secret, the scales fall from our eyes and the way to success seems so much more achievable.

It has nothing to do with superior brain power. Studying this program, if I can call it a program, is so simple it will, once success has been achieved, make it seem like common sense, just as a champion tennis player makes the game look so easy. Should that happen, by then you will feel like a champion and start to taste the benefits of a changed life.

This is what this book is designed to do, and hopefully people will respond to it and experience a difference in their lifestyle. By beginning to look at themselves in a different light, appreciating what an amazing, miraculous creation the human body, mind, and soul is that they have been blessed with, life will never be the same again.

This new life comes with a responsibility to be cared for and looked after. When, it prospers so will you. Unfortunately, due mostly to ignorance, not being able to see the wood for the trees, so many folk stumble along living a humdrum life. These are the people, the ones who are still caught in the trap of mediocrity, I would like to reach and show that they can also enjoy some of the better things life has to offer, who have not yet realized what they are capable of, and the fact they are also important. Just think for a moment the difference that could make to the lives of so many folk with a diminutive perception of themselves. Let's see if we can be successful at snaring their attention in a simple and light-hearted way.

It is common for many people who come across any subject they see as even slightly challenging to sidestep and avoid it like the plague. That is the main reason behind the thought of putting it across in as light-hearted and simple a way as possible.

The idea is to create the impression of a group sitting in a circle while discussing the different subjects, with me answering their questions.

Everybody is frightened of old age and the unknown. That should spur the not so young on to get a look in a little further than where they are at the moment.

The idea is for the individual to understand that looking after the mind and the body is by no means a drag, but can be and usually is great fun and cause for enjoyment. When that happens, the soul automatically follows suit, and when all three are liberated, incredible results and gains will automatically follow and their objectives achieved in a way that is not tantamount to experiencing purgatory.

In the beginning, it may be a little difficult, depending on age, physical condition, level of motivation etc. Once past that point, it is downright fun all the way. To prove that not everything worthwhile in life needs to be difficult and serious, a lot of light-hearted pleasure was had writing the book. Hopefully, that will become obvious while reading it, at the same time emphasizing the enjoyment that can be experienced while taking part in the different exercises, and revealing what enormous positive gains can be enjoyed by eating better and living a more sensible lifestyle. It is my purpose to make them understand the end results can be hugely rewarding and be great fun at the same time. There are no lectures, just guidelines the reader will find very easy to follow, the kind that everybody can understand once they have been made aware of how easy it is. Life can be incredibly beautiful. Is that not what it was meant to be?

BOOK ONE

Introduction

DREAMS

We all tend to daydream at times, young and old. Most of the realistic ones can be realized when we adopt these suggestions in this proposed way of living, not only for a fortunate small percentage. The average person who makes up by far the largest percentage of the population, as well as the better-off, and those who are not in very good physical condition, perhaps already down the line to a miserable old age, can still enjoy a dream that life could be better, more active, full of fun and enjoyment.

For many it remains just that, a dream. Reading this, hopefully they will realize there is light at the end of the tunnel. There is always room for improvement and great benefits, in spite of past experiences, disappointments, conditions, and circumstances. In other words, the dreams are dreams no more, they are becoming a reality.

For the majority of people who allowed their free will to take its course without any active interference on their part, resulting in a state of dismay and unhappiness, or even worse for many of them, there are ways to bring about a change. Many who would like to change the quality of their lives on their own, often do not see their way clear to making a start, simply because they lack the courage due to the fact they do not know how to or where to begin.

While the percentage of active people are increasing all the time on account of the attention the holistic way of life is enjoying at the moment, there are still a huge number who believe that luck has passed them by and they will never experience what it is like to enjoy a physically active life. In the same vein, there is hope for the many people who because of some disadvantage in life feel inferior and do not believe in themselves. In the section on the mind and discipline, motivation is dealt with and they will find the help they need.

Ninety percent of the population falls within the average bracket. A small percentage (call it five percent for argument's sake) are gifted in some way or the other, or are of above-average intelligence. On the other end of the scale, we have the people who are mentally or physically challenged, approximately also five percent. That means that the likes of you and me must fall within the ninety-percent bracket.

I am aware of the fact that life is never that simple, but also not as difficult as it is made out to be generally. There is hope for most of those unfortunate folks who still hold on to the dream of an active lifestyle, but feel they have left it too late. Just take it easy and go at a slower pace. Everybody can fit in somewhere in the program. In the case of doubt about any condition, consult with your physician and if he declares you not within any danger zone, go for it – there is a way to a ***better life and a happier you.***

Starting at an early age holds distinct advantages. In the financial world for instance, in the category of life assurance, the younger you start contributing to a scheme, the less you pay to achieve the same amount at the eventual pay-out. As you get older your contributions become bigger. Unfortunately, not pro rata. The latter is several times more expensive in order to achieve the same financial benefit in the end. Although of a different kind, this is also life assurance for the physical, mental and emotional side of life. It is of equal value and works in the same way.

If you are young and perhaps not in a good physical condition, it is so much easier to keep going along the same old way year after year. Unfortunately, although you can do that, your physical condition will deteriorate at a much faster rate. Before you realize what is happening, in real terms you will be ***ten*** years older, while unfortunately, the body will be the equivalent of ***fifteen*** years older due to physical deterioration caused by the weakening of the body tissue. Muscles remain strong only if they are stretched and exercised. It is so much easier to make a firm decision to take care of yourself from as young as possible and apply the brakes to avoid physical neglect.

In a young adult person, the body tissue is new, fresh, vibrant, and it is much easier to maintain the physical and mental quality you are enjoying at that time than to build your future from there. The longer the delay, the harder it is to play catch up and salvage some quality of life.

When you reach a certain age, say past the half-way mark, to reverse the deterioration is distinctly more difficult, but not impossible. Perhaps it will not be a hundred percent turn-around. That depends on age and condition, but any improvement at any stage of neglect is a big one. The tissues will show signs of wear, and the veins and arteries may be clogged with cholesterol, but don't despair. Lots of vitamin E plus vitamin C, as well as lots of second class (vegetable) protein, plus a little exercise, can improve the situation.

We have only one life. We pass through here but once, so make the best of it. The rewards for making an effort to improve your life are enormous – you owe it to yourself and your loved ones, and even friends and acquaintances will notice and feel good for you. *There is not a single life on earth that can't be improved upon with a little effort,*

A person consists of three divisions: mind, body, and soul. All three must receive treatment in equal measure (known as holistic). If any one of them receives scant attention, the whole person suffers. We are a finely balanced entity, just like the universe, the earth, and life itself. Should the balance be disturbed, chaos ensues. It all adds up to discipline. We all know some person who has neglected **the** most important mission in life, which is not paying enough attention to his health (mental as well as physical). Most of the time, we look after the mental side very well by achieving a good education. On the emotional side, we fall in love, get married, but unfortunately do not care for the physical side with equal enthusiasm.

It is a great advantage to continue with physical activities directly after finishing school and not fall into the trap of "taking a gap year." Continuity if at all possible, should not be interrupted. This is the time where young people should show a certain amount of maturity. It is not wise to think of old-age as being a long way away and will look after itself. To spend the last ten or fifteen years of your life at ten or twenty percent throttle is the time you and your doctor become very well acquainted, usually at enormous cost you can ill afford when you should be enjoying your old age. This does not add up to a whole lot of fun – overweight, pain in the legs, no energy, certainly no enthusiasm to be active.

You can experience the exact opposite, playing with the grandchildren and sharing an active lifestyle with them. Otherwise, you not only deny yourself a lot of pleasure, but also the grandchildren suffer, who own the right of attention and pleasure from their grandparents. This is an aspect of life that is noticeable in many countries where family units are very important and the grandparents play a huge role in the upbringing of the grandchildren, resulting in a strongly bonded family and a stable and happy society. It is not only desirable to maintain an active lifestyle from a young age, but also very much easier to maintain a positive outlook with all the benefits that will ensue.

This is not meant to be just another book on health, or a general idea on what to eat or not to eat, and what is good or what is bad for you, although it may seem to be so at times. The idea is to bring to the reader's attention the importance of a holistic or partly holistic way of life, with all the benefits that can be enjoyed.

If the idea of a holistic way of life sounds too much of a change to even think about, relax. It does not matter what percentage of a holistic way of life you adopt. Even a small percentage can make a difference to your general well-being. The general intention is not to make a holistic way of life sound like it is equal to a prison sentence. Far from it.

It is not what you do occasionally that does the damage. There isn't anything wrong with feasting occasionally. *It is what you do on a regular basis that matters and sets the trend that determines where your life_will take you*; either a rocky path that is disguised and appears to be smooth but ends in disaster, or a holistic way of life that may seem to you to be a really difficult mission, almost impossible to manage.

There are many ways to achieve results. Fortunately, there are easy ways and more difficult ones. This one you will find to be one of the easier ones, guaranteed to achieve tremendous results rapidly, simply because it is based on an *effortless natural way of living.* Even if it may seem totally the opposite at times, the way to live should ideally be as natural as humanly possible. We *are* natural beings after all. To achieve success, we can but do one thing only, and that is **cooperate with nature as far as possible. The joy of success will far outweigh the effort.**

My motto, generally speaking, is to keep it simple, get back to basics, do not complicate matters (which makes it difficult to see the wood for the trees), and don't look for a complex solution to unravel a simple everyday problem.

Life is not as complicated as we tend to think it is, or as it is made out to be. The intention is to show you in a simple, interesting, and fun way how the body and all it contains work. All too often a person would consider the body and what goes on inside this mysterious creation and think, "This is not for me, leave it to the experts." Unfortunately, the experts do not live in your body, you do, and it is your responsibility to become better acquainted with it and your life in general. No one else can do it for you.

You will find it not at all difficult to understand the way the body works as this is presented in simple terms, and you have some fun while being introduced to a fascinating subject that concerns us all. You will find very few scientific names and titles. Leave that to the professionals. Once you have read the book, hopefully a small flame of interest will have been kindled on the subject and a much wider desire to know more about the workings of the body, which will no longer be a scary subject.

Perhaps a completely new direction of interest, even an exciting new hobby is waiting for you, with huge benefits. (An interest in your health can indeed become a new hobby. That is what happened to me). This will far outweigh any other you may have had in the past, and is definitely far more important, for instance, than finding out about vitamins, minerals, salts, sugars, and acids, the actual food of the body. Let's forget about them individually and refer to them by their cumulative term – nutrition. What they are, the functions they perform in all the different organs, the skeletal system, the blood, nerves, and much more.

Every part of the body needs not only one but several different forms of nutrition, and often some of the same items are found in different organs in different combinations. Sounds complicated? Not at all. You do not have to remember many of them, only the ones that are important, and they are few enough not to be confusing. This information is mentioned merely for interest's sake to let you know the choices that are available to you. The material to get to know them is available but not essential to digest, to have a healthy mind, body, and soul with a wonderful lifestyle and enormous gains.

It is disturbing to notice how careless people are about what goes into their mouths, almost treating their bodies as rubbish bins. Such lack of respect towards this miraculous creation we were presented with, almost always leads to disastrous consequences during old age or even earlier, which could have been avoided. What is so difficult to understand is that very few people realize they are responsible for the sad state of affairs and simply accept it as their natural destiny. A common remark is often heard, "my dad was overweight," as if it is natural for the offspring also to be overweight, an easy way to sooth the conscience by shirking the responsibility for one's health.

See the holistic way of life as a good friend. Perhaps it will take some time to get to know him, but it will not be as difficult as it may seem. Follow the steps one by one and absorb all the good advice at an easy pace. The end result will be absolutely astounding. Good friendships do not come cheaply. This one will be well worth the sacrifice and is usually for life.

I know once you have been captured by this friend's charm, there is no way you will want to separate from him. Nevertheless, a negative attitude is subtle and can easily become part of your life again, even though you do not want that to happen. Be on your guard at all times. The old habit, the one you left behind, is not a willing loser and will try and trip you up on a regular basis. Remember what life was like before.

Look towards the future when you make a decision, particularly the far distant future – the latter years of your life. Yes, they are as important, if not more important than those you enjoy right now. A healthy old age starts when you are in your prime and your body is still strong. Old age can last a long time and if you are not prepared when the time comes, it can be very hard and difficult. On the other hand, it can also be great fun. Make the choice for the better. Aches and pains, and even worse, are not fun and games when your life is past its prime. It should be a lot more fun and certainly can be, if you are prepared when it arrives.

Life is slightly cockeyed. You grow up, and when you are least qualified you are supposed to choose someone to live with for the rest of your life and raise a family; then you have children when you, once again, are least equipped to do so; then you grow old and should you follow the route most people do, with the "really don't care" attitude, you will live to regret it bitterly with the excuse that there was nothing you could have done about it. It does not make good sense not to care.

This is not the time to be in poor health, full of aches and pains, resulting in lots of visits to the doctors at a time one can ill afford it. Financially, it is much better to spend your pension money, which is usually a lot less than you earned while still employed, on more enjoyable activities. A huge bugbear is inflation. Pensions do not get bigger, they tend to get smaller. Medical costs increase and medical cover shrinks. If you are not careful, this leads to sitting in long queues at some government hospital, hardship when you least can handle it. The answer: ***take control of your health while you still can by living sensibly.***

The usual plan for when you are on pension is to travel as much as possible. The question is, will you be fit enough to enjoy the wonderful places you want to see, even if you can afford it? Travelling can be physically demanding. Following a holistic way of life you are, bar accidents and the like, guaranteed to be full of energy, ***the envy of all, to enjoy your old age.*** Yes, it is fun to be seen as fifteen years younger than people of your own age.

My interest and enthusiasm to know more about nutrition was acquired in my early twenties. Although I was an avid reader from early childhood, my love for books on health matters came about in a rather unusual way. As an enthusiastic sports person from a very early age, consequently extremely fit and healthy, it was really bizarre that I was laid low with severe bouts of "flu" as regular as clockwork, several times a year. What was the cause? Nobody knew and even fewer people could figure out what the problem was, or the reason for this unhappy state of affairs. After many professional medical opinions, one even said I had a virus on the lungs and needed a course of injections. Who knows what he pumped into my body, all to no avail. How this poison affected poor hapless me who had no say in the matter of my well-being, I will never know. Well, I survived, thanks to the incredible resilience of this wonderful creation, the human body.

That was then the subject of good health caught my attention, and I subsequently developed an interest in nutrition. During one of my frequent visits to a bookshop, I came across books by the great dame of nutrition, Adele Davis. That whetted my appetite for more knowledge on the subject. Little did I realize at the time what an enormous influence on my life this visit to the bookshop would have over a long period of time, as a matter of fact for the rest of my life. The influence it had on my thinking as far as nutrition and eventually my eating habits were concerned, I would realise only much later when I began to see the extent to which people, including myself, take good health for granted and the careless way we abuse this incredible creation, the human body, we have been so blessed with and privileged to live in. The attitude we have, that man lives to eat rather than eat to live, with appalling results, became so apparent in my way of thinking, that a new determination was born within me to be different. It was inevitable that my way of life, and eventually my life as a whole, would never be the same as I saw happening around me.

Cautious optimism becomes part of life when we venture into uncharted waters. It was no different in my case and it took a while to reach the information concerning milk. What a revelation that discovery was to me. I grew up with the indoctrinated idea that milk was essential to growing up healthy and strong, and then to learn that the opposite was true. My love for and obsession with milk was to blame for my regular illnesses. Erroneously we were told to drink lots of milk to give us strong bones. Why we needed such incredibly strong bones is to this day not quite clear to me. We are not beasts of burden and what we have is adequate for the sports fields. Hallelujah, I was so much the wiser to discover how detrimental to good health the use of raw cow's milk really is, and that there are other forms of nutrition much better suited to the purpose of doing what cows' milk is supposed to do. Further on this subject will be handled in more detail.

My regular visits to the sick bay were at an end. It was not an easy task. It was difficult to give up such a deep-seated habit. That led me to another of my wonderful discoveries – mind control, which obviously did not happen at the same time. That sort of maturity does not happen overnight. One grows into it unless one is shown the ropes, which makes things a whole lot easier. Mind control will also be handled in detail later on and made much easier to understand (chapter 12).

My idea is certainly not, and I must stress this, to put any doctor or the medical profession down in any way whatsoever. I have the utmost respect for doctors, they are wonderful people. In my entire life, I have not had the experience of meeting an unpleasant or arrogant physician. That certainly is noteworthy. What the medical profession has achieved in the last few decades is mind-blowing. What once took an enormous incision and a long stay in the hospital now happens during keyhole surgery and one overnight stay in hospital.

What has become known as "keyhole surgery" is now a daily occurrence and we are fortunate to live in this era. Unfortunately, the cost of medical treatment has become horrendously expensive, and one cannot but wonder where it will lead to when governments will not be able to bear the cost and medical aid schemes become so expensive that the ordinary citizen can no longer afford medical cover.

My interest in the workings of the human body and mind just kept on growing. It has always disturbed me to see how uncaring the average person is towards this miraculously designed and incomparable machine, the human body.

The reason for people's reticence to be more concerned about their health, in spite of so many warnings, continuous rhetoric, professional advice, books written on the subject, and endless television programs, is hard to understand. The public's blasé attitude remains a mystery. It seems the general public has become so adapted to the idea of a physical breakdown in the human body that it is "normal" to have something ailing you. Could fear of the unknown be the reason? This reading should change all that. The body, human and animal for that matter, is so near to perfection there is simply nothing to compare it with. Looking after our health should be our first priority, even if it is out of sheer gratitude, let alone our duty towards our maker.

It would be so much cheaper for the government to supply the less privileged citizens with fresh vegetables via some scheme or the other. That will save billions on building endless number of new hospitals and training staff, as well as supplying costly medical aid to keep the population healthy to put right what went wrong in the first place due to a lack of nutrition. I suppose this will remain just a voice in the wilderness. The body is so designed that should one care for it in a proper way and eat the food designed for its

maintenance. Bar accidents, one can to a large extent with a few unfortunate exceptions, expect it to keep operating in a normal fashion to a ripe old age.

These were the reasons that motivated me to do this writing. To try from a different point of view to get people's attention and show them how marvellous their bodies are and how they should pay a little more attention as to how they treat them, and perhaps develop a new or deeper interest in the maintenance thereof. Yes, *maintenance* is the correct word. Staying healthy does not happen automatically, unless the person has been raised with that objective in mind. It is shocking to see how little the average person knows about wholesome nutrition.

Highlighting the finer detail of the body and the workings thereof, hopefully, will grab the reader's attention and set him/her off in a new direction to a new rewarding self.

This is a difficult one. Which came first, the chicken or the egg? Education on the subject should start at the earliest possible stage in a child's life, **preferably** before the child can form his/her own opinion. **When children reach that stage, the taste for good nutrition should be a part of their lives.** I was witness to a perfect example. Two children, three and four-year-olds, were offered some sugary sweet/candy. The words and wisdom that came out of one little child's mouth was remarkable. "My mommy said we mustn't eat sweets, it's not good for us." Guess who were the more enlightened of the two, the parents or the adult who should have known better, but did not? Let's not be too harsh but put it down to a lack of interest, an all too common attitude.

If parents don't know how and what to teach their children as far as nutrition is concerned, the horrendous statistics that stare us in the face daily will only get worse. I cringe when I see a mother hand her child a packet of potato crisps, a stodgy, oily, object completely devoid of any nutritional value Harmful? I would say so. Let's analyse the offending object. Taste, before it was camouflaged with myriad colours and flavourings, was bland and unattractive. Then it was treated with commodities containing artificial additives, which are designed to stimulate the taste buds. Motive? Profit, no thought spared for the well-being of either the parents or the children. It will more than likely have several ingredients that could be suspect. Monosodium glutamate and the colorant, Tartrazine, are additives that are banned in many countries, but unfortunately not all. For convenience and the sake of profit, the use of these hideous substances are widespread. I was witness to a perfect example to see the effect Tartrazine has on children.

A friend came to visit with two little children, and while strolling along the beachfront the children spotted an ice cream parlour. The inevitable happened. Two ice creams of their choice were bought, deep and dark in colour. The effect this had on the children after consuming the ice cream was remarkable. Before they were normal lively children, afterward they were completely out of control. Mother did not notice the difference. It happened all the time so to her it was "normal."

Imagine the effect this must have on the nerve centers in the brain where the effect is registered. Prolonged use of this offending chemical, like a myriad other chemicals people dishonour their bodies with in the name of convenience, taste, and pleasure, is completely alien to the well-being of the person, and totally out of character as to the design of food for the human body, which is not equipped to process chemicals that are not of natural origin. Hopefully, you will find interesting what is in the offing further on and enjoy a happy healthy lifestyle.

Life does not start when we retire, not next year or in five years' time, not even tomorrow. The rest of your life starts today or better still, right now, this very minute. This is the first day of the rest of your life. Life is an ongoing experience from birth to the end. It does not take a break at some time or another. Parents look at the little miracle in their arms with great expectations and unmatched intentions... exactly the right food, the right amount of sleep, the right amount of emotional attention. Why, so meticulous? Otherwise, the human race may not have survived as well as it has, or definitely not optimally and we would be short-changed throughout our entire life. Unfortunately, good intentions are most of the time short-lived. Unless a special mental note is registered, memories will fade pretty fast and the good intentions are good intentions no more. Would it not be a good idea to maintain the same meticulous attention and reap good results for the rest of the child's life? Does that make sense or not?

Psychologists will tell you the best time to start the human race off on a good habit, or any habit for that matter, is from birth to five years, the impressionable age. That is the time when the human computer is empty and waiting to be filled with whatever it is presented with, unfortunately, good as well as bad. The subconscious, where all material the mind needs to operate is stored, is highly impressionable. It takes very little input to make a big impact, with some good fortune. For instance, becoming aware of the fact there is a much better alternative lifestyle that could be followed.

Whatever is absorbed mentally, or the child perceives at that age, remains there for the rest of that person's life.

To raise well-adjusted, happy children and eventually adults, can be relatively easy by paying attention to what is allowed to enter that young mind before age six.

THE BODY

Chapter 1

TOXINS

With lots of love, good nutrition, firm discipline, and strong emotional guidance, the first five years of a child's life will ensure a reasonably easy time for parents during the rest of their childhood and beyond.

Parents take note, for your child to be successful, not only physically but mentally and emotionally as well, is relatively easy as long as the above is applied before the age of five. What is allowed to be registered in that little mind is important. As with the positive aspects, when we make sure the child develops abhorrence for anything that is not of any benefit, will be registered in that little mind and that thought will become part of that child's personality for the rest of its life. I can testify to that statement being true. My father made sure I understood from early childhood that cigarettes are diabolical objects and smoking the filthiest habit one can acquire. I still hold on to the same sentiment to this day.

We, including every component in our bodies, are natural creations, and this happened long before the word science was ever thought of. Very often as a matter of fact, by far the majority of times when things go wrong in the body as a result of consuming unnatural substances included in the modern diet, it is possible to make a correction by following a more natural way of life.

We all make mistakes one time or another. *Modern diets can and often do create problems with dire consequences that will manifest much later in life. Natural science then has to come to the rescue, if it is not too late. One is not always aware of the alternative, a more natural diet. I will endeavour to introduce you to this wonderful way of life*

Many impressive sounding scientific names have been invented for many detrimental consequential conditions that occur when a body has been badly neglected and abused, mostly due to ignorance. Many of them could have been prevented. During the repair process, we should not isolate a certain condition or treatment. The body is a holistic entity and should be treated and maintained holistically as a single unit.

It is wise not to stint on the quality and quantity of natural food. By doing that it is inevitable that you will be spending a lot of time with your doctor at enormous cost later in life. The difference: In the end, the quality of life is expensive and below par. On the other hand, eating natural food is so much cheaper. Due to the much higher nutritional value, you consume so much less in comparison. The end result is a much better quality of life.

The body is not designed to get sick. By far, the majority of illnesses are caused by eating what we should not eat, and not eating what we should eat and those of psychosomatic origin.

We are what we eat. Detoxing is the buzz word that has held center stage for quite some time. Unfortunately, many people do not quite understand what it means. What is detoxing? It is merely removing poisonous substances from the blood which has been contaminated by an excessive amount of toxin (poison) present in a neglected digestive system.

All foods leave toxins behind. The toxicity found in food varies tremendously from natural raw foods with very low toxicity content which the liver and kidneys can easily take care of, to the "don't care" attitude to eating anything simply because it is "nice." The way the body was designed to operate, compared to the "rest" which is virtually anything eatable, often with a high toxicity level – one could be realistic and call it poisons – is detrimental to the maintenance of a healthy lifestyle.

Although the body has a natural ability to remove toxins via the kidneys and liver which will be explained at a later stage. How it happens is not relevant at this stage. The statement above will suffice to understand basically what toxins are, and how we can help the body rid itself of these undesirables. I would just like to mention that the body has limitations in its ability to handle the task of keeping itself clean on the inside, and it is our duty to lend a hand when we are careless or overindulge on food that lacks nutrition too often.

This chapter is designed to make it easy for the lay person to understand what toxins are and how to rid the body of this scourge and maintain a healthy standard of living. Right now, it is a buzz word that most of us don't understand. The process is very simple and nothing to be afraid off. The commercial world is right up front and charges huge amounts to do the detoxing for you (a horrendous process), and absolutely not necessary. There is a more natural way, free of charge.

There are two systems operating within the body. One is the digestive system. This is where the toxins are formed. The second is the vascular system, which becomes contaminated with the excess toxins the liver and the kidneys cannot cope with. It consists of the blood, blood vessels, and all the related sections of the vascular system. Detoxing refers to cleaning the vascular and digestive systems.

Present-day standards and way of living is not a commendable method to achieve optimum energy levels, longevity, and general good health, on account of the high levels of toxins found in the body of an average person on a modern diet.

The ability the body possesses to rid itself of toxins is probably at maximum efficiency when we are children, although even at that age the body is not capable of doing the job by itself, should we over indulge. As we get older the body becomes even less efficient at performing sanitation on itself, and every year the efficiency level drops.

At middle age, it is well down on efficiency, so bear this in mind when next time you hear, "I don't have to bother, I am regular and my kidneys and liver do the job for me." Not true, by far not efficiently enough on account of the fact that the average person is not particularly concerned as to what goes into their bodies. That puts an enormous demand on the filtration system (kidneys and liver). The body is amazingly resilient, and to a certain extent it can cope with, shall we say, "Foreign matter," food the body is not designed to handle. Unfortunately, the accumulation effect makes it impossible for the body to stay in a clean and healthy condition.

Do not lose sight of the fact that the body is primarily designed to handle only natural and organic foods. It is also true that the way we prepare our food kills off a vast amount of nutrition and natural fibers, resulting in a high percentage of waste material. Remember, anything dead deteriorates rapidly, more so in the body where ideal conditions exist for such a condition to develop, like temperature and moisture, with a fair amount of artificial **chemicals thrown in for good measure.**

Just pause for a moment and consider some of the many chemicals, foreign to and absolutely incompatible with our metabolism (which is natural), we consume on a daily basis. Amongst others are commercially produced preservatives, emulsifiers, stabilisers, colorants, flavourings, white flour, white sugar and too much salt etc. etc.

The body is not capable of removing all the toxins, so what is left over stays in the body and the problem increases progressively. It needs some help, and that is taken care of by the "toxin removing food" we should eat.

These are, for instance, fresh vegetables eaten raw where possible (delicious recipes do exist and this will be discussed later), dried fruit, and the most important item, lots of fresh fruit (of which the nutritional and substance values have always been underestimated by the layperson), and adequate quantities of water.

Also recommended would be an occasional *blood cleansing herbal product (e.g. stinging nettle). Use a crushed level teaspoon-full in a glass of boiling hot water, allowed to cool and taken at bedtime.*

At first, take it every second evening for one week, then once a month. Make sure to ask for the dried herbs and not the tablets. These are available at your local health food outlet, as well as many pharmacies which should be able to help you. But allow me to stress that the best and most natural way is still via the fresh raw vegetables and fruit routine, with the cleanser once a month.

The herbal cleanser will do the same for the digestive system. In the event the herbs are not available in your area, ask for anything similar. It must be a blood cleanser. Some that come to mind and are more or less universally obtainable are Swedish bitters, Cascara, Lemongrass, etc. My personal favourite is Stinging Nettle, which cleans both blood and the digestive system.

A daily glass of Lemongrass tea, or Redbush (commonly known as Rooibos tea), is a simple and easy way to achieve the desired result and should be part of the daily diet. The folk in many rural areas in underdeveloped countries who, in spite of maintaining a reasonably healthy diet, maintain a custom to obtain the same result still in use today. They take extra precautions on a regular basis to maintain a healthy digestive system, for instance, drinking sea water. I would not recommend or approve of taking sea water (salt content). This is only one example. Every tribe or nation (usually underdeveloped) has its own way of dealing with the situation.

As children, we were administered a dose of Epsom salts and I cannot recall ever having suffered an infection of any kind. In this modern day and age, such an idea would not go down very well, but it is imperative that the inner body is kept clean for optimal function ability, as well as to prevent infections. Yes, believe it or not, infections.

Allow me to throw a cat amongst the pigeons.

Keeping the body clean on the inside to prevent infection makes a lot of sense. Should an injury be sustained, infection is created from the muck that exists in an unclean system when it comes in contact with germs from the outside. If the body was clean on the inside, the natural immunity that exists in a healthy body would be able to cope with the onslaught from the outside and be capable of preventing infection from setting in.

Germs are not the all-powerful enemy they are made out to be. The body is well equipped to defend itself against these enemies, provided it is not hampered by compromising conditions that form on account of neglect, not always deliberately; most of the time it is simply ignorance.

If we were to believe the outrageous advertisements on the media, should the all-powerful and all prevalent armies of germs on the war path looking for an opportunity to strike be true, the world population would have been wiped out by now. It is common knowledge that the world is overpopulated by a vast degree, apparently by 50%. As far as the advertisers are concerned, the terrifying germ armies are prevalent everywhere, ready to unleash their all-conquering might and wipe us all off the face of the earth. To prevent this imminent disaster is the equally powerful deterrent, a simple bar of soap all to the benefit of the great gods, money, and profit. Not that a bar of soap, (read the chapter on soap and skin) would be able to keep infection at bay in the case of an injury to a body with a compromised vascular system. A clean vascular system would not need any help, not even from an all-powerful bar of soap as the advertisers would make us believe.

To be so over-protective towards ourselves and our loved ones is not a good idea. We are all aware of the natural immune defense system all bodies possess to start with, provided it has not been interfered with. By fighting the "presumed" excessive unhygienic conditions and ridding the environment around us of "all" germs, to the extent that we become neurotic, can compromise that very important natural defense mechanism.

Give the system a chance to strengthen itself and provide the body with the opportunity to defend itself against attack. With a more naturally nurtured and stronger immune system, there is much less chance of contracting a condition detrimental to the well-being of the system.

Most of us in the community I belong to are ardent travelers. One particular country that is a very popular destination has, unfortunately, the reputation that you go there with the foregone conclusion that some time or another you will fall ill should you sleep in anything less than good or expensive hotels. When a friend was asked the inevitable question about his well-being while he was there, he answered that he took precautions before he left home. And what were they? His reply was that he strengthened his natural immune system by, for instance, not washing fruit and vegetables before eating them, nor washing his hands unnecessarily, etc. etc. I do not expect parents to become reckless, but do maintain a level-headed attitude.

I was standing behind four delightful young ladies, obviously on holiday from school. We were on an escalator in a large shopping center, and I was thinking to myself how beautiful youth is, happy, not a care in the world, excited at what the day of freedom would bring, when one girl innocently put her hand on the hand rail. The other promptly removed the young lady's hand, pointing her finger in a fashion as to explain the danger of such a reckless move. It was not difficult to deduct what the lecture was about. Our minds no longer belong to us. We have been completely sold down the river by the advertising moguls all in the name of profit. I don't for a moment think that the welfare of the nation is of uppermost concern; to them it is merely a matter of mega profits.

There is another very important reason to avoid toxin build up and potential catastrophic conditions forming in the body, which has been neglected for a long time, perhaps having never received the attention it deserves. In many cases where the toxin build-up is severe, and the person suffers an injury, where treatment could have been a simple matter of attending to the wound and allowing it to heal normally, now it becomes an emergency with infection setting in, and medical attention becomes necessary or at least alternative treatment, which usually includes antibiotics.

In cases where antibiotics had been administered often, a certain amount of immunity has built up. The fear that antibiotics are in danger of becoming irrelevant due to their overuse, is well known. As far as I am concerned, the use of antibiotics should not be taken lightly by anybody who follows a healthy lifestyle. Provided the external conditions at the time of the injury are not unhygienic in the extreme, their bodies will be able to cope with any mishaps that occur under normal everyday conditions. Obviously, should an accident occur under extremely unhygienic conditions, the necessary precautions should be taken, but first observe if the patient is coping or not before administering antibiotics.

Kidneys are hardworking organs in the body with an unenviable job to do. Although they are resilient little fellas, they are, after all, designed to handle only food that is natural. It is nothing less than fair that we assist them in every way possible when we are inclined to abuse our bodies by living recklessly as far as what we eat is concerned. If only we knew a little more about what happens inside our bodies concerning this subject, especially the kidneys, which is really not difficult. My motto: **Keep it simple**. So, read on.

The following explanation will be sufficient for the lay person to understand why the body should be treated with a whole lot more respect than is the case on average. The attention we see around us concerning the subject is motivated by fear more so than common sense. It goes without saying that the well-informed and sensible person will make an attempt at adopting a more responsible attitude.

We were born with two kidneys and can survive very well with only one, probably with good reason. They are so important it is only relatively recently that kidney transplants became possible. Please do not think that it was your destiny to receive a kidney donated by some kind-hearted donor. It could more than likely have been averted.

Bear in mind that kidney dialysis is a dreadful consequence of not only failing to pay adequate attention to what we eat and drink, but also not paying the necessary attention to maintaining a healthy lifestyle in general.

Kidney dialysis has become far too prevalent in this day and age. I am not referring to kidney failure where individuals were born with malfunctioning kidneys, or reasons other than kidneys that have deteriorated on account of neglect, which far outstrips the first mentioned, i.e. their owners not paying enough attention to what they consume or to the maintenance of their kidneys by regularly **removing toxins**.

The practice of detoxing has become a very large industry. The emphasis is placed on the magic word "Detoxing" and big money is charged for the service.

The sad thing is that folk are brought under the impression that "it's done now and I am OK." That may be so, but should the lifestyle remain the same, all the good work will have been in vain and it will not last very long. It is essential that the emphases is shifted to where it belongs.

Detoxing should be part of our eating regime. The body should be kept clean on the inside at all times by eating correctly and taking an herbal cleanser at least once a month, as well as taking the aforementioned tea daily.

Poor choice of diet and quantities the body is not designed to handle are the culprits.

The occasional binge will leave you none the worse for wear. It is what we do on a regular basis that matters. The Bible equates gluttony with drunkenness. If you are a person who is reasonably concerned about the state of your health, but a little doubtful about what you are reading, make an effort to speak with someone who is undergoing dialysis treatment for diabetes or broken down kidneys, or see the process in operation, then perhaps you will be of a slightly different opinion and realise what you are reading is true. Even to the extent of visiting a hospital to see first-hand, it is that important. On the other hand, many individuals accept it as "normal, just one of those things" that sometime during their lifetime it may very well be an unavoidable part of life to experience such a traumatic event.

They either do not know better, or don't understand that the state of affairs is not normal and the situation could have been averted. Imagine how different that life could have turned out to be, perhaps many more years of healthy living.

It is imperative that we take an interest in our own well-being, and realize it is our duty to gain some knowledge on how the body functions and make an effort to maintain it.

A very dear friend, an old lady, of sound mind and still very much up-to-date on what was happening around her, chose death rather than continue with the dreadful and painful treatment (dialysis). Yet it is avoidable in the vast majority of cases. It is our duty to be more circumspect about our lifestyle. We do have choices to make. It is our responsibility to make the right ones or pay the price.

Should the kidneys show signs of deterioration, a temporary "mainly fruit" diet together with an herbal cleanser should be adopted immediately. Fruit still remains the most beneficial food one can eat. It is also the best antioxidant by far. The juice in the fruit purges the body of all undesirable elements. In other words, it assists the kidneys in ridding the blood of toxins. Fruit will also help lighten the workload of the kidneys and give them a chance to heal themselves before a more natural diet is followed. To say that they will recover completely may be possible depending on the condition they find themselves in, but it may just avoid that dreadful possibility of dialysis or even worse, a kidney transplant. There is no reason why a much longer fruit and raw vegetable only diet could not be adopted. Should this route be followed, to prevent constipation it is important to go easy on soft fruits like pears etc. Some acidic fruit should be included, and a slice or two of "whole wheat" bread would be recommended. The herbal cleanser can be taken more frequently. Do persist, it will take some time for the body to become regular due to the change in diet. Once it has reached normality, it is plain sailing for as long as you stay with the good habit. The difference will be mind-blowing.

Don't be alarmed if your urine suddenly becomes darker when you eat a lot of fruit, when you thought it should be a lot cleaner and consequently lighter in colour. What actually happens is the abundant fruit juice is doing what it is supposed to do, purging the body of toxins and that is the only way the toxins can be expelled from the body.

Should you become a little constipated on a fruit diet, make stewed prunes a regular part of the diet. Also, eat a large handful of bran flakes at breakfast time. Half a glass of fruit juice will also help to relieve the situation. Natural yogurt washed down with some water should be taken before every meal.

After a course of antibiotics, it is of the utmost importance to take a substantial quantity of probiotic. The reason for this is that antibiotics are designed to destroy bacteria. In the process, the good bacteria are destroyed as well. Natural bacteria are vitally important for the digestion of food and should be returned to the stomach as soon as possible. Pro-biotic can be bought from any health food store, as well as many pharmacies that have seen the light and have taken to stocking a large variety of natural products.

While we promote the use of natural products, the Almighty is always a few steps ahead of us. He has been doing it for an awful long time so let us keep to his recipes. A natural product He designed for a natural purpose is yogurt, an excellent natural pro-biotic; not the flavoured kind, just ordinary, natural yogurt. The human race's taste buds have been high-jacked to such an extent that it cannot tolerate anything edible that has not been flavoured, sweetened or salted.

Refer to the chapter on the mind and learn that it takes only a small amount of time to get used to a new flavour and better still, enjoy it.

Once your mind has been trained and it has been convinced and sold on any new idea, it will rebel against abuse once it has been converted to the new thought and taste of a positive nature.

Once your taste buds have been restored to their natural condition (with the help of a reformed mind), it is amazing how downright tasty natural yogurt really is. You would not want to go back to the artificially flavoured kind again.

You may have heard via advertisements that some yogurt (like many other foods) is flavoured by natural products, fruit for instance. I am convinced that the few pieces of fruit in the product are **not** enough to alter the taste to the extent that it does. I am convinced there is also some artificial flavouring present, but on account of the fresh fruit, it can be claimed that it has been flavoured with fresh fruit, with the artificial flavours mentioned in type so small that it is hardly possible to read.

Do not forget, the body is a natural entity and natural building material should be the desired choice. People in the know will tell you that it is possible to artificially manufacture almost any flavour, be it fruit, vegetable, honey, or any other kind of edible commodity.

In a badly neglected body, the healing process may be so restricted that healing cannot take place fast enough, and the infection can often move into the bone and cause one could lose a limb. More severe cases of toxin overload can prove even more problematic after major surgery, when it becomes a huge battle to get the body in a condition to heal itself (a process only the body can perform). Natural cell forming, and more infection-fighting ammunition is needed in a desperate effort to save a life or limb, often to no avail. Now is the time to become convinced of the merits of adopting a more responsible attitude towards our health and well-being by reverting to a more natural lifestyle.

Visiting a neighbour to see how he was doing after surgery, I was quite shocked to see the wound, the stitches bulging with puss pouring from every little opening. Although he was trying to show a happy face, I could see he was desperately ill. I left to fetch some herbal remedy I always have on hand to remove toxins from the body and gave it to his wife with instructions for him to take before he went to sleep. I did not visit him the next day but the day after, and it was pleasant to see that he was looking and feeling so much better.

The sensible thing for me to do would have been to suggest more of the same treatment. I still remain convinced that it would have been the right choice to save his life. In a case of that nature, one has to use discretion, not jump in at the deep end. Legal ramifications could be severe, taking into account there was a physician involved. One could speculate whether that was the right choice for me to make, to my way of thinking and if it were possible, it would not have been a difficult decision. Sadly a week later we buried him at the young age of fifty-nine. Apart from the poison that eventually caused his death, his body was still in pretty good shape, a young age for a person to pass on, and so unnecessary.

Where ideal and healthy conditions are present after surgery, and all the necessary nutrients, right conditions, and material that are needed for healing are available, as is the case in a healthy body, it stands to reason that healing, which is an ongoing process, will be so much faster. After all, no human effort can heal any medical condition, only the body can heal itself by rebuilding the lost, broken, and damaged cells. Medication can perhaps provide comfort, but it cannot heal the body. Sometimes people die long before they should, not to mention the inevitable suffering that usually precedes death. That could have been avoided had the person known about keeping the inner body clean in, which case the healing process simply would have carried on doing what it normally does, and do best – heal the body. *Infection always starts from the inside of a neglected body and not the outside as is so commonly accepted.*

One can compare the reaction that takes place when infection occurs to that of a catalytic one. The bacteria from the outside has to combine with the unclean conditions on the inside to create an infection. When healthy and clean conditions exist where an injury has occurred, the natural antibodies will be able to fight off the bacteria which tries to enter into the body and minimal interference to the natural healing process would be necessary, perhaps just cleaning and dressing the wound.

Healing, which is an on-going process will take over. The tiny little cells will just keep on forming and multiplying, like they always have done; multiplying and growing, every cell in its appropriate place to repair or form complete new tissue. The healing process is rapid, and never stops. It is a never ending, an on-going process every second of twenty-four seven.

Severe pain is caused by infection, mainly by the pressure caused by the chemical action that takes place while the infection is forming, and the stress caused to the surrounding tissue. After surgery or an accident, it is notable how quickly the patient with a clean vascular system recovers.

Recently meeting up with a lady friend I had not seen for some time, I noticed a severely swollen index finger (almost twice the size of the other fingers) that looked very unhealthy, inflamed with a yellow hue to it, a sure sign that it was severely infected. Apparently, she had a slight accident to her finger. A fish bone penetrated between the nail and the cuticle. That happened nine weeks earlier, and several visits to the doctor later, and in spite of taking several courses of antibiotics, things did not look good at all. Guess what? My old favourite came to mind – herbal treatment.

I suggested she take the blood cleansing herbal remedy that starts work immediately by removing toxins from the body, including the spot where it is needed, via the blood that transports it from the intestine, where it was received after the stomach and intestines performed the function to perfection. It is a natural product formulated by nature for the purpose. Five days later I called on her to find the finger still slightly swollen, but looking decidedly healthier with a much-improved colour and well on the way to being normal again.

Recently I was paid a backhanded compliment by nature. I discovered a hairline crack on top of one of my molars, but I was not in a hurry to have it seen to as it felt small and was hardly noticeable. Sometimes I wondered if it was perhaps my imagination. It was there, in a big way (never underestimate the sensitivity of the tongue; think about that for a moment). Once the dentist got through the hard enamel on top, he discovered a huge cavity. Enquiring why l had left it so late, l explained that I did not know that it was there, and was asked about the pain. My reply was that there was no pain, which was hard to be believed by both of us, a strong sense of skepticism was noticeable. The inside of the tooth was completely gone and required an enormous amount of rebuilding.

After three visits, l asked his professional opinion regarding the lack of pain. The only explanation he could suggest was that I have an unusually strong immune system. *I never told him my secret. Does it bear out my statement that pain will not occur in a body with a clean vascular system because infection was not possible?* We all know what toothache is like and how dramatic it can be. Moral of the story: keep your body clean on **the inside** and the chance of infection and pain is so much smaller, or none at all.

A lady friend had a brain tumour removed. Although the procedure was successful, after several weeks the wound was still weeping puss. She accepted the suggestion to use the herbal cleanser and within a week it was so much better. Within two weeks it was completely healed. What made the difference? The toxins were removed.

Once again, it explains how much easier it is for the body to do its maintenance and rebuilding work when the work area is clean and there is nothing to hamper its efficiency and progress, compared to the condition of the average body that has never experienced the luxury of being purged of the enormous toxic build-up over many years.

Think for a moment about the resultant conditions of the enormous variety of food and also muck we eat that could not possibly be called food the body has to cope with. When this variety of material is thrown together, chemical reaction and toxin-forming are almost instant, the body's natural cleansing system (mainly kidneys and liver which purifies the blood) cannot cope on their own. It is not designed to handle the enormous volume of unnatural material.

The saving grace lies with the fact that the body is remarkably resilient. It will cope, sometimes for very long, but will eventually throw in the towel, unlike a clean well-kept body where everything works extremely well and natural maintenance takes place automatically.

No organ, tissue, or whatever is not in prime condition, can cope with toxin density so high that sufficient tissue maintenance is not possible. The intestine walls cannot contain the leaching or seepage of toxins, which eventually end up in the bloodstream and then onto the rest of the body tissue. From where it travels to every nook and cranny, like the joints between the bones, etc.

I cannot substantiate my theory, apart from conviction from personal experience and advice that turned out to be successful to others, that these toxins (which are more like poison by now) can be responsible for causing all sorts of problems, for instance forming crystals that lead to many different maladies that originate from inside the body. Arthritis comes to mind, which is just one of many.

Alzheimer's, yes the dreaded disease that sends shivers through the mind of those who have had the unpleasant experience of witnessing someone so unfortunate to have suffered this dreaded condition.

Alzheimers is a condition where there is a chemical present in the brain that slowly erodes some part of the brain. Where did this chemical come from, and what prevented the brain from doing what it should be doing naturally and that is to repair the damage as it happens? My response (for what it is worth) would be that the body was so overloaded with toxins that it could not respond and was prevented from doing what it was supposed to do. My second thought would be that the chemical was the result of a long line of stray chemical reactions, as would happen in any laboratory (the body) on account of the toxin overload. Consider the potency of the chemical, which is no more than a drop in size, in this tiny tablet is capable of subduing and influencing the brain of a grown man. The mind boggles.

Could chemicals that react directly on the brain tissue (which is of a very delicate nature), like headache tablets or tranquilizers taken over a long period of time, not have a bearing on the forming of the disease? Perhaps the answer lies with researching the medical past history of the victims as well as the disease.

What could be the cause that makes so many bone transplants such a necessity in this day and age? Perhaps toxins that form crystals and have become so severe that they attack and break down the bone tissue in the joints?

Hopefully, this will set a train of thought in motion that sometime somewhere in the future may lead to further research. It does sound like an extremely simple solution to a very big problem. According to common perception, life is never that simple (or so we are made to believe). Could it be that the answer to the problem was too simple to be noticed and was consequently overlooked in the process of finding an answer? My preferred maxim: *"Keep it simple at all times."*

Think about this (following the statement above): If there are no toxins, material that creates infection on the inside of the body, there cannot be any chance of infection. Should the skin be broken, for whatever reason, the resultant strong immune system will be able to handle any attack that comes from outside. It goes without saying the same will happen deep inside the body as well.

l would like to suggest that in cases where maintenance to the digestive system is an on-going process, by eating correctly and paying adequate attention to proper maintenance, it will be possible to do away with antibiotics altogether after surgery. It will be a tough decision for a surgeon to make. (It has been discovered that the hospital is the most dangerous place when infection is under discussion). Close observation will probably do the job of playing policeman, and the decision made to only then administer antibiotics when deemed necessary. An ideal situation? If only life was that simple.

Am I against antibiotics altogether? No, not at all – the invention of antibiotics has proved to be a huge blessing to mankind. It is a tricky situation. One cannot expect the physician to gamble with a patient's health. Rather, it remains the responsibility of the patient to make sure the hygienic condition of his body is of a sufficiently high standard to keep the amount of antibiotics to a minimum should it become necessary for them to be prescribed.

These would be ideal conditions to live with. But, could the same not be said for the painful conditions that are so prevalent such as rheumatism, arthritis, kidney problems, and a whole host of others?

As suggested above, are these conditions not caused by waste and chemical products which are deposited in the joints and then form crystals that make life such a painful experience? Should one be able to avoid these crystals from forming by keeping the blood clean and free of any toxins, would it perhaps be possible that the problem could be minimized or completely prevented from occurring? An acquaintance complained about pain in his wrists which had not yet been diagnosed as arthritis. My suggestion was that he switch to this new lifestyle with nothing to lose as it may just work. He accepted my advice and the pain in his wrists disappeared completely. Spare a thought for all the curtailed suffering that could be realized with the possibility of research proving that these thoughts have merit.

Another friend of long-standing told me about the pain in her wrists she has to endure daily without let-up. Feeling great sympathy for her, I suggested she take some blood cleansing herbs. After all, that is where the muck in the body is to be found. I saw her some time later and asked how she was feeling The answer: a whole lot better. Every moment when possible, my life is spent out-of-doors where the chances of suffering injuries are ever present. Scratches from rusted wire were a regular occurrence, as were scrapes from branches, barnacles, cuts, and bruises. I watched friends being treated with the appropriate remedy, but always declined the offer when it came my way, and never had a problem with infection. I can't say the same for them, in spite of taking preventative action.

Imagine if we could see inside the body, specifically the digestive system and we had X-ray eyes that could magnify hundreds of times. There we would find these tiny cells and their helpers in a neglected body full of toxins. These poor little fellas would be slaving away under atrocious conditions, totally exhausted making minimal progress, trying to move this bulk of virtually useless nutritional material through the digestive system, having very little to pass on to the blood whose job it is to supply the cells with building material. The heart that has the unenviable job of moving the blood through arteries that are gunged up with cholesterol, is slogging away twenty-four seven at a heart-wrenching seventy-five or more beats per minute. No wonder at some time or another, it simply gives up the fight, and we have a heart attack to deal with. What a waste of a God-given life that was meant to be enjoyed.

Now look at the opposite scenario. A clean on-the-inside body, where our little fellas are singing while they work, smiling from ear to ear, as fit and as healthy as their owner, full of energy. They have hardly any work to do. The nutrition from fresh raw fruit and vegetables glide through the intestines without any obstacles in their way. The abundant nutrition pours through the walls of the intestines without effort into the blood, flowing through clean arteries, richly laden with every conceivable form of nutrition, happy to deliver this to the cells that gorge themselves on the lovely loot. The heart strong and healthy, does not know what hard work is, pumping away at a leisurely pace of fifty beats per minute. Their owner has so much energy, thinks clearly, sees better, all the senses on permanent high alert, enjoying a fantastic way of life. Is that not what it was all meant to be?

Something to think about: why is there so much wrong with the human race health-wise? In spite of the obvious affluence, the better off countries are always the worst affected. Here we are not including the very poor who simply can't find enough food to eat, but still finds the means to acquire the food that will keep them healthy.

Consider the number of transplants that take place every day. Making these components and marketing them has become a multibillion-dollar industry. What is the reason for this? Is it possible that God had such a huge preference and love for wild animals above us human beings? The reason I mention "wild" is that domestic animals are as prone to getting sick as often as their owners do.

Wild animals, on the other hand, provided they never come in contact with humans or suffer accidents, with few exceptions, are born, go through their allotted period of time on earth, and then die without ever getting sick. *Why compare us with animals?*

A simple reason: the difference as far as DNA is concerned is only 3-5%. There is only one possible answer and that is the incredible amount of disdain we show towards the well-being of our precious bodies.

Add to that the enormous burden the economy is lumbered with. Medical insurance has become expensive on account of the high cost of surgery and hospitalization. Once again, "Lord Money" reigns supreme. These institutions and individuals have the human race over a barrel. Greedy to fill their pockets to bursting is no problem to these folk. For them, there is no such thing as having enough, regardless of what that means to the potential financial ramifications for the population as a whole.

Medical procedures and hospitalization are already so expensive that medical insurance cannot foot the bill, and the insured, in spite of the fact that he pays his monthly contribution, is held responsible for the balance. The portion he has to pay is often the equivalent of several months' income, which leaves the patient with serious problems. Eventually, governments will have to foot the bill, with money that simply is not available. Will the situation become so dire that sometime, somehow, the human race will come to its senses and live with a little more common sense?

It is, after all, a joy to live with an attitude of respect towards life. The benefits are vast, not only financially, but on every level of consciousness. It is all simple, positive, and so rewarding.

By now the reason for spending so much time emphasizing the importance of keeping the body clean on the inside should be quite clear. Stodgy food results in a stodgy body which equals a stodgy lifestyle, and all the losses that go with it; very little or no energy, resulting in a lack of interest in life altogether.

The victim of a wasted life is always aware of this unpleasant bit of information long before it becomes a crisis, but on account of ignorance does nothing to rectify the situation until it is too late. There is just enough time to rue the fact that he/she did not treat their God-given health with more respect.

Cancer: there are many different forms of cancer. Many have been dealt with it successfully, but sad to say many have not. Is it not our duty to do our utmost to prevent, wherever possible, contracting this disease by keeping to the manufacturer's natural maintenance plan?

A well-run waste disposal plant is usually clean, respectable, and relatively odour free, while the site that is not well-run is diametrically the opposite. Every person has his own little waste disposal unit and it is just as important that we run our lives along the lines of the first-mentioned, and reap the benefits accordingly.

It is imperative that we visit the toilet once a day. Toxins multiply alarmingly fast and should be contained in the area provided for that purpose to stop an overload from spreading to the organs and other parts of the body via the blood stream.

Perhaps the resultant damage to these organs in the short term may not be noticed. Allowed to multiply, the deterioration in the quality of life, no matter how small, will soon be noticed by an alert person. That level of alertness should be the target for everybody to achieve.

The evidence of poor nutrition is often noticeable. Constipation would be a certain indicator that all is not well. Unpleasant smelling bad breath is usually the first symptom to be noticed by bystanders. Bad smelling perspiration and then passing winds is usually a dead giveaway. A remedy for the interim would be to take a regular dose of herbal cleanser (dried herbs and not the tablets) at least once a month or taken as directed. Once a balance has been achieved and you eat lots of fruit and raw vegetables when possible, life should be noticeably more comfortable. No need to wonder if the smell of your breath or body is noticeable and offensive.

A simple test to determine the state or degree of cleanliness on the inside of the body is to wear a shirt for only one day. Hang it outside the cupboard and check the level of the odour under the armpits in the morning. The level of odour present should be an indication of the level of toxins present in the body. No toxin no odour. To be a hundred percent sure, it is recommended that no soap be used to wash the body (read the relevant chapter on soap and skin).

Can too much be said about toxins? In my opinion, the answer must be no. Another product that produces a lot of toxin and worth some attention is Plastic.

The word plastic is actually a misnomer in the English language. Plastic is a French word meaning to mould. The correct word in English is synthetics. There are many different kinds of synthetics, each with its own individual characteristics and purpose. Some are soft, some hard or tough, depending what the particular purpose they are intended for. The different products are made by combining different chemicals of the same kind in different combinations to form the different products meant for various purposes, a process that was first invented in the early eighteen hundreds although it took all of the next hundred plus years to give us the products we enjoy the use of today.

It is very important to take the utmost care when you store foods in synthetic containers, particularly liquids. Some of the chemical components are less stable than their counterparts and could release chemicals that will contaminate the food. This contamination may be negligible, but over a period of time could reach significant proportions that can cause detrimental consequences to one's health.

Many of us have had the experience: "I don't know what's wrong, I just don't feel well, but the doctor can find nothing wrong with me."

It is often not easy to diagnose a condition without the aid of extensive blood tests being carried out, usually at enormous cost and several visits to the doctor. Could that also be a contributing factor to the premature aging process, in other words, the general degeneration of the body tissue? I would think so. The toxins or poisons that accumulate in the body over a period of many years cannot produce good results. The body is forced to spend an enormous amount of energy combating the onslaught of that which are actually more than mere toxins, but in actual fact chemicals.

The body's amazing ability to resist these poisons can hold off the onslaught for a long period of time, until the proverbial dam wall bursts and we start to feel the effects of poisons manifesting themselves in various ways. Then it is time for drastic action on the medical front, often to no avail. The negative effects do not end there. The normal positive repairs, rebuilding, providing nutrition, a process that takes place in the body continuously, is also hampered and cannot produce its best effort just to keep us alive.

There is one brand that is least destructive and is acceptable as far as the people in the know are concerned, and this is polycarbonate, used widely to store a wide variety of soft drinks. Polycarbonate is a hard product compared to other synthetics and can be recognized by the crackling sound when it is squeezed. It is deemed safe for storage of many liquid products and purposes around the house. It will be hard to manage without this versatile product that has become so popular, but not impossible. Glass, ceramics, earthenware, or any product from natural material should always be the first choice.

We are not the only ones that have had to suffer the fate guinea pigs do. Two thousand years ago during the time of the Romans when lead was first used in the manufacturing of water pipes and also in glazes during the manufacturing of ceramic food and liquid containers, many people became very ill, and even died, before the reasons for their demise were discovered. Lead used in the manufacturing process was to blame.

Chapter 2

DIGESTION

Why does digestion demand so much attention? Digestion begins in the mouth. When the food is not masticated properly, for one, we can suffer indigestion. This means the stomach receives unprepared food. Consequently, it cannot do what it is meant to do, process and prepare the food to allow the nutrition to be extracted. Therefore, the acids and chemicals cannot do what they are designed to do, fulfill their natural functions, which are to create nutrition to feed the cells which, in turn, perform maintenance work on the body. Wherever discipline is interfered with, chaos ensues and the stomach is no different. The following is the way things should happen under ideal conditions.

First, we chew the food in the mouth where it is mixed with saliva, a very important digestive juice. Saliva is a major component of the digestive juices. It is essential that we chew our food very well, at least thirty times per mouthful. Yes, you heard correctly when your teachers accentuated that point at school and they were not being facetious. Our stomach does not have teeth. Saliva, a digestive juice, is squirted into the mouth to liquefy and pre-prepare the mixture, resulting in an extremely fine paste. Should food not be broken down properly while chewing you will miss out on nutrition that is trapped in the remaining roughage of even the smallest particles.

From there it is moved down to the stomach by means of the peristaltic movement, where it is mixed with acids and other digestive chemicals. This is where the digestion proper takes place and the food is prepared for the nutrition to be absorbed into the blood stream.

Now it becomes clear why it is so essential that food is finely mashed while still in the mouth. The finer the better, even small crumbs matter which contains nutrition, this is a very delicate stage in the whole digestive process.

The vitamins, minerals, salts (not table salt but the natural salts found in the food that we eat), sugar (again not refined sugar but the natural sugar we find in our food) acid (natural) and vegetable fats are formed during several chemical processes from the different foods that we eat combined with the chemicals in the stomach. All the different nutrients come about only after the chemical process has been completed. We do not take vitamins and nutrition by mouth, they are the end result.

The stomach is a very complicated laboratory. This is where the mixing and processing, together with the help of a large number of different chemicals, take place. Only when this process has been completed is the mixture moved along to the intestines, where only the nutrients are absorbed into the blood through the walls of the intestine. The first part of the intestine system is called the small intestine, except there is nothing small about it. It is meters long, but there is a reason for it to be long. This is where the absorption of the nutrients takes place, a slow and complicated process. One should not rush the eating process. The more time we allow for the digestion of food the more efficient will the whole process be **which is so essential for good health.**

There are no mechanical or physical means to separate the nutrition from the rest of the food. It all happens by a process similar to "osmosis" (easier to understand). That explains the reason for the enormous length of the small intestine. From there the nutrition is transported by the body's unique transport system, the blood, to every single cell in all the different areas of the body where it is needed to build, repair or reconstruct (for instance after suffering an injury). The repair work is an on-going process, twenty-four seven, it never stops. This process provides energy and oxygen to the muscles, without which we would not be able to move, and all the other purposes that require nutrition. For instance, building an immune system, creating all the different chemicals the glands require, bile that is needed to digest fats, and many more. The list is enormous.

If that is not amazing enough, the small intestine is divided into three sections, the Duodenum, the Jejunum, and the Ilium, and each section takes only the nutrition it has been designed to remove from the mixture. For instance, several vitamins are removed by the duodenum, another group by the jejunum, and the protein is removed by the Ilium. Some really fancy design work, enough to make any scientist green with envy. When it reaches the end of that particular line, the end of the small intestine, all the nutrition that can be used has been removed and the rest is no more than mere waste and is moved into the large intestine or the colon, not much more than a storage space, ready for evacuation.

I have often heard the remark, "why don't you eat more solids?" Mistakenly it is generally accepted that the body absorbs solid foods like meat for instance. No, all that is absorbed in solids like meat are chemicals, for instance, amino acids before it is converted to protein. But unfortunately, what is detrimental to good nutrition are the animal fats that meat contains (creates cholesterol). Meat is also highly toxic. The toxicity varies widely in meat, red meat being the worst offender, then chicken, white meat, and fish, which is probably the safest of the animal proteins.

Saliva is more than just water. It is a complicated mixture of water and chemicals that mix with the chemicals in the stomach to prepare the food for digestion. Considering the fact that digestion begins in the mouth, it becomes clear why it is important to chew our food properly and *we do not drink water* while chewing our food, provided the food is not too dry, in which case a little water taken with discretion should do no harm. The water dilutes the digestive juices. Drinking some liquid, with discretion, after it has been swallowed is the answer.

The importance of the amount of saliva nature allows into the mouth while we chew the food can be noticed when we brush our teeth. At the next opportunity when brushing teeth do not rinse the brush, only apply toothpaste. After the wash, check how much liquid is in your mouth. Another reason for the need to drink adequate volumes of water regularly during the day is to remain hydrated, especially during the warmer months. Premature aging is partly attributed to the lack of moisture in the skin.

The blood needs a constant supply to maintain a desired level of viscosity, and to prevent cramp during strenuous exercise on warmer days (there are other reasons why muscles cramp as well). The recommended quantity of water is approximately six to eight glasses per day. That does not mean water only, all liquids are included. It will certainly do no harm to drink more liquid. Eight glasses should be the minimum for a person who maintains a sedentary lifestyle. The quantity should increase together with the increased activity. More on this subject later on.

Indigestion is the repeated abuse of the digestive system. In the chapter on nutrition, it will become clear how one should treat the digestive system and its different components with the necessary respect to maintaining a healthy lifestyle. The occasional feast should not cause any discomfort in the digestive system. It is constant abuse that is the culprit, like eating foods that are not designed for consumption continuously. The body can handle these conditions to a fair degree, but sooner or later it will start to object.

To lend further assistance to our digestive system, take a few teaspoons of natural yogurt a few minutes before every meal, then wash it down with a small quantity of water. This will create new bacteria that will mix with the bacteria already in the stomach to form a formidable force to handle the task lying ahead with ease. It is also a powerful weapon against constipation. (Only a top quality, heavy bodied unflavoured yogurt should be used).

CONSTIPATION.

While on the subject of digestion, allow me to say a few words on the subject of constipation. **Where there is a hindrance of free-flowing movement in any of the highways and byways of the body, eventual problems can ensue.** The bowl and colon is an area that is frequently overlooked. Constipation should be dealt with instantly. Neglect to do so can lead to serious medical problems, followed by major surgery and even death if not attended to. The moment the condition develops treat it with blood cleansing herbal products or a mild laxative. Herbal products should be one of the favourites in the kitchen.

ADEQUATE WATER INTAKE IS OF THE UTMOST IMPORTANCE TO AVOID CONSTIPATION, AT LEAST SEVEN GLASSES OF LIQUID PER DAY.

Chapter 3

NUTRITION

Consider fresh vegetables among many others, for instance spinach, which has a beautiful colour. Colour is very important, not only for aesthetic reasons but it is a good indication of the nutritional value present in the vegetables. When they are vibrant, crisp, just begging to be eaten nutritional value is almost 100 %, depending on the freshness and the length of time since it was removed from the soil. Is that important? Yes, but not critical. Vegetables can last a number of days after harvesting. Put in water for a while and they can then be stored in the refrigerator for the next few days without losing too much nutrition. Ideally, the vegetables should be stored in plastic bags in the refrigerator with the oxygen (air) removed as much as possible, and the vegetables will last considerably longer with most of the nutritional values intact.

Now let's look at the same spinach after having gone through the cooking process (by the way spinach is arguably one of the top most nutritional vegetables we can eat). Imagine what it looks like after it has been cooked – a lifeless unappetizing blob on the plate. Sure, condiments, flavouring, colouring (often with artificial ingredients not welcomed by the metabolism will be tolerated in small quantities though not recommended in the long run). Natural ingredients, which should always be the first choice, can be added to make food more enjoyable. The artificial additives will not restore the destroyed nutrition. The fuel, the building blocks that the body needs to grow and reconstruct lost nutrition to ensure a long healthy life full of vitality, fun, adventure and a great future depends upon **adequate nutrition for optimum health and boundless energy.**

Creamed spinach does make the mouth water – nutritional value, very little if any. Man cannot live by bread alone, and what is the sense in living if we are deprived of delicious mouth-watering creamed spinach and the like occasionally? There is nothing wrong with a bit of occasional decadent culinary indulgence. It is not the occasional decadence that matters, the body can easily cope. What we do on a regular basis is important. With too much rule-bending the system will put up a brave front, but will eventually start losing the battle and with it a healthy existence. Mouth-watering dishes can be prepared from fruit and raw vegetables, even raw spinach, with a little imagination and creativity. There are many recipes and publications available on how to prepare delicious dishes from raw ingredients.

With holistic thinking well established, together with myriad holistic cookbooks that are available, there are literally hundreds of delicious recipes to choose from. A little stretch of the imagination, even one as poor as mine when it comes to food preparation, can perform wonders. Just imagine a mouth-watering Smoothie, all the nutrition intact, delicious ripe fruit prepared with lots of fertile imagination. Think how much fun you and your loved ones will have on a rainy Sunday afternoon. Once you experience the benefits of eating proper food, there will be no stopping you expanding your repertoire, and the kitchen can become an exciting place to spend a lot of free time experimenting as you begin a **completely new direction into what can become a very interesting new lifestyle.**

It will not be long before the change within yourself will become obvious when the little cells are better fed on wholesome food, loaded with adequate nutrition. The healthy little cell, together with billions of other cells like him in the same organ, turns that under-par performing unit into a vibrant active one. The same happens to all the other organs, the brain, the eyes, all the muscles, blood, and so on. Consequently, much more energy and more interest in life results. Physical improvements include clearer vision, skin tone and colour changes, losing weight, altogether a new you with new interests in life.

Is that not enough reason to spur one on to make the effort to improve one's health and continue on a successful quest to a better lifestyle?

After all, you pass this way only once. One may as well make the best of the opportunity, all at no more effort, but a whole lot cheaper on account of the fact that one eats much smaller quantities because of the higher nutritional value and volume (weight loss). It is important to eat the right food to guard against malnutrition. *(Yes, the correct word, even well-fed people can suffer malnutrition if too many nutritional components are absent).* It pays to be vigilant and look after that side of the bargain as well, the well-being of those precious little gems known as nutrition.

It is not only overeating that has become a big problem with the wealthy section of the world; equally important is the lack of a healthy diet. With a healthy diet, the food has so much more nutrition. You automatically eat less and weight loss follows naturally. What you neglect to eat and should eat is as important as eating what one should not eat to maintain optimum health.

Nutrition, yes that's what it's all about, the be all and end all of a life that is lived to the full; or the opposite, an existence that is a drag, consisting of commuting from the one object of rest to the next, motivation and energy levels at rock bottom, preferring the easy chair to anything that involves moving of any sort. Far too often it leads to being overweight, and a negative frame of mind, and low self-esteem. These are choices we make continually, often without even being aware of doing so. Even not making any choice could also be a choice we make, often conveniently to bypass the guilty conscience.

Sometimes we do so knowingly, irrespective of the consequences we are well aware that will follow. Is that ignorance, not being aware of consequences or an "I don't care" attitude? Often both, I guess, accepting the status quo as inevitable and believing that kind of life is destined to be our lot. There is good news with lots of opportunities to move on to a much more interesting lifestyle. *(At this stage it is important to include reading chapter 18 on losing weight together with this chapter to learn more about the importance of eating more fruit and raw vegetables).*

All those smart asses out there, and believe it or not the majority tend to hold on to the ridiculous "I don't care attitude," only until some time later down the line, when everybody is expected to pray for them. God helps those who help themselves.

Imagine the opposite: a family that one way or another were made aware of the wonderful opportunities available out there, grabbed it with both hands and used it to spectacular effect to better their lives, full of energy, bright-eyed, lean and healthy. Naturally, their minds would be keen and alert, they would have endless energy enjoying recreational activities, bounce off a chair as if spring-loaded instead of having to use the armrests to lift themselves, walk briskly instead of dreading the prospect of moving at all. Is the last mentioned what life is meant to be? I don't think so. ***Amazing how often the result of that attitude is assumed as their lot in life. How does one change the situation?***

Easier than you may think. Ever heard of "it's all in the mind"? Very true, it's all to do with attitude. The mind is easily manipulated as is explained in Chapter 12. Read more on how the mind can and should be manipulated in a positive way to achieve our goals (to be read at a later stage). Once the mind is convinced of the relevant facts, it will understand how to bring about a change of attitude leading to a vastly different lifestyle. At that stage, it is the trained mind that will do the directing when you want to stray from the golden path you have chosen. The going gets considerably easier as we go along. To make the first positive move is the hard part. From then on it is a new adventure, a new interest in life resulting in a completely new person.

Looking at human bodies, the neglected and the well cared for, we do not notice any obvious difference apart from the one looking healthier than the other, but what goes on underneath or inside the skin is a totally different story – the many different organs, skeletal system, nerve system, the way it all fits together, works in tandem, each organ, muscle, bone, down to the tiniest cell, all in the exact position it was meant to be and performing the function it was designed to do. The difference in performance and end results are huge.

It all begins with the tiny body cell we are all familiar with. It is amazing what takes place inside that minute entity and how it works. Every cell is a living little miracle, completely self-sufficient when it receives the necessary attention. Every cell needs nutrition, food to sustain itself, to grow and multiply as the body requires new material, the building blocks to repair damages to body parts as well as replacing dying cells which happen on a never-ending basis.

Neglecting the nutritional side of the bargain, not supplying the necessary nutrition the cell requires, the health and well-being of that cell will deteriorate, even die. Should that happen to too many cells, the body begins to suffer and this soon becomes obvious to ourselves and those around us. We put on weight, we become sluggish, we lose our energy and eventually we lose self-respect and interest in life itself.

Every organ and the cells that belong to that organ requires its own variety of nutrition peculiar to that particular organ, its own vitamins, minerals, salts (not sodium chloride or better known as table salt), sugars (natural, as it appears in food not white or refined sugar), fats, acids, all natural. For instance, the skin would need vitamin A, D, the nerve system vitamin B, the arteries vitamin C, the blood vitamin E. Naturally these are not the only vitamins and minerals each body component requires. It needs a combination of several with the ones mentioned of primary importance (more on this particular subject at a later stage).

It may seem like huge amounts of nutrition are needed to keep the body in prime condition, but fortunately, that is not so. It is amazing how small a quantity will keep the body in tip-top condition. Perhaps not a large amount in physical terms, but large in variety. The quantities are minute –consider the size of a multivitamin capsule where one finds most of the nutrients present. Not that one can live on vitamin capsules alone. You still need enough food to satisfy the requirements and demands of the body to function with all the nutrition present.

It is important to see vitamins in the correct context. Although only supplements to the food we eat to ensure a proper balanced diet, they are vitally important to the diet as will be gleaned from this discussion.

Allow me to mention something that has been widely accepted. Nutrition contains the building material the body needs to create cells, and for that reason they can also be seen as a "medicine." In other words, the repair work they do is known as natural healing. *As we eat ourselves sick by means of neglect, we can reverse the process and eat ourselves well again by eating food rich in nutrition.*

Apart from the combination of vitamins any particular organ needs, it is of dire necessity that one takes a considerably larger amount of the main vitamin that is needed for any under-par condition. For instance, vitamin C to keep the arteries in good condition or to help arteries in poor condition to recover, vitamin E to keep the arteries free from cholesterol, or vitamin B for nerves in poor condition, than is prescribed by the R. D. A. (recommended daily allowance which is meant for a healthy body to stay healthy) which has been the same for more than fifty years that I know of. Perceptions and research have changed enormously during that time. There has been an explosion of knowledge a million times more accurate than in the past, thanks to modern day research, new innovations like computers and the like. Quantities will be discussed in more detail later on as well as the importance of not going overboard.

To know which foods supply the correct vitamins is a subject important enough to warrant the time and energy required to read books on that particular subject.

The importance of this writing was not to create a new book on nutrition (many have been written over the years and are as relevant today as they were when first published), but rather to create an interest in a subject of mammoth proportions and undoubtedly on the most important choice you will ever make, *the importance of natural nutrition.*

Now that your interest on the subject has been kindled, I hope you find as much joy in pursuing a new lifestyle and finding the correct reading material as I did when I first started my quest for better nutrition. Not that my health was ever challenged (apart from drinking raw milk during my youth), far from it, subsequent improvement to my nutritional intake, I believe, made a huge difference. There is always room for improvement, or maintaining a good physical and mental condition. It is so much fun, and the rewards will far exceed your expectations. It is bound to change your outlook on life completely once you have established a new interest.

The following is purely my own effort at varying the menu by making a Smoothie of high nutritional value. It can be simple, basic or can be downright delicious. The principal purpose of this recipe is to have the biggest variety of ingredients made available to the body. As you go along you will understand how little nutrition we really need to be healthy, so use just a tiny portion of each vegetable and fruit to taste. This creation can be very rich in taste, start small.

A Smoothie is still the easiest way to eat raw vegetables with delicious fruit juice, which is the secret. MOTHERS, a definite and easy way to persuade your children not only to eat their vegetables but eat them RAW, not only delicious but with several hundred percent more nutritional value free of charge. Save on your food bill by using much smaller quantities due to the fact that they are eaten raw. Vary the taste by using different fruit juices and ingredients.

HOW TO MAKE A SMOOTHE

Start with a half-cup of fruit juice diluted with water to three-quarters full. In the blender, add half the ingredients finely diced by **putting the leafy ones (spinach) at the bottom.** What is to follow is very important. The machine must run as short a time as possible Switch it on, hold on to it tightly and shake it gently. As soon as all the ingredients have been sucked to the bottom, turn it off. Alternatively, divide the quantity into two portions. **The final product could be rough allowing for chewing to be mixed with saliva, or allowed to become a paste (mushy, not too appealing), in which case it should be mixed well with saliva before swallowing.**

Compare the quantity of ingredients to what you are used to in the cooked variety. A cup full of spinach, after being cooked, has shrunk to about a quarter of its size. Nutritional value is probably no more than 10% of the original, considering the heat and boiling water treatment, which is certainly not gentle on vitamins in particular and nutrition in general. For instance, roughage is completely destroyed.

Compare the Vitamin value of the two. Raw 100% (depending on the freshness, which is the same in both instances). Roughage also 100%; after cooked 10%. One has to eat so much less to receive a huge increase in nutritional value. **After all, that should be the main reason why we eat,** though fortunately not the only one. Eating still remains probably the most enjoyable pastime that ever came man's way. I will not argue with that. I love eating good and delicious food. What is good food though? The choice is huge and variety still remains the spice of life. Once your sugar craving taste buds have been re-educated and have been restored to what they should be, or the way they were when you were born, you can also experience the joy of tasting what natural sweet, unprocessed, and uncontaminated flavours are really meant to taste like.

Experiment, it will be a whole lot new fun and so much healthier. After a meal, you do not feel like keeling over on the bed and going to sleep. No matter what your age, you are full of energy and feel like asking if anyone feels like taking a stroll. What is missing? The heavy bulk of dead food sitting in your gut weighing you down and causing you to want to go to sleep so it can create enough energy to get on with a lost cause – digesting that bulk, *in which case most of the energy in the body is used to digest the food we eat.* Rather use the energy doing something positive and productive or while having some fun.

As a matter of interest, while on vacation recently I climbed Table Mountain, a well-known landmark in my country, without stopping once and not in the slightest out of breath when reaching the top. It is not very high but at age 75 I think it is worth mentioning to prove a point. Eat your vegetables raw.

For my Smoothie, check what goes into the blender: Any vegetable that can be eaten raw, even the ones you may think not suitable to be eaten raw may be used, but concentrate on a variety of colours. Experiment with different combinations until satisfaction is achieved. (This and a raw salad are the only way to eat vegetables).

Fruit Smoothie: (Begin with a small portion of fresh fruit then add to taste). Any strong tasting fruit is a good choice. My favourite is grapefruit, orange, or pineapple. Fruit is a very powerful food rich in nutrition and very much underrated. One can live off fruit alone (a subject that should be well-researched before embarked upon). I still prefer to eat fruit the natural way, with a knife.

Now for my vegetable Smoothie:

Any number of the following vegetables (not the sprouts)

- Three or four leaves of spinach (not the spine).
- One small carrot or part of one.
- One segment broccoli.
- A few sprigs of parsley.
- A slice pepper, any colour, preferably green.
- Sprouts from three or four different seeds.
- A five mm thick slice of cucumber.

- A small celery stick.
- A small tomato (or part of one).
- You can use any vegetables you wish to.
- A small sized spinach or Swiss chard leaf, or two or three or more, highly nutritious, the blood builder, lots of iron and protein. This is a highly nutritious ingredient. You can virtually detect the difference between the before and after use. The small variety tastes better.
- A small handful peas and the same for beans (frozen will do).
- Add some fruit like orange to enhance the taste.

Sprouts can be made at home or can be bought at the supermarket.

Important: the mixture must be consumed immediately. Reason: oxygen destroys vitamins. The action of the blender sucks in huge amounts of oxygen.

This will make a fairly large glass of health drink, contains all the vegetables you require, and taken daily will be sufficient to keep you on the right track to a healthier you. Should it become tedious, try and vary the ingredients. Not a huge price to pay for a vastly improved lifestyle, lots of fun, energy, and vitality. Be patient and experience the best.

This alternated with a salad can or should become a standard procedure. Vary the ingredients at will.

Cooking food that does not need to be cooked is a waste of good nutrition. Do remember to swirl the mixture in the mouth to mix with saliva, which is a very important part of the digestive juice before swallowing.

HOT RAW SOUP

Yes, your eyes are not deceiving you. Something entirely different and equally nutritious and delicious, it can be made from the ingredients above with some modification to suit soup. Use most of the ingredients used for the Smoothie and if you prefer, add some boiled potato to vary the texture. Leave out what you think will not go with a soup recipe, and add what appeals to you. Add boiling hot water to the mix in the blender, just enough to cover the vegetables. For taste, add some vegetable stock. Go easy, some brands are loaded with salt. I use a portion of a spiced vegetable patty, only a quarter of one patty for one serving soup, or to taste. Absolutely delicious, and a whole lot healthier than the average commercial product. Do not forget the sprouts that are a little old and long in the roots, which are still highly nutritious. As for the nutritional quality, the raw soup is a huge improvement on the cooked variety, still 100 %, added to that the fact that it is also hot.

Use cold water should you feel like cold soup. You can make any one of the cooked soups with cold water. (One very important point, use only freshly prepared vegetables). Avoid the prepared soup mix ready for cooking. The vegetables already prepared could be a day or two old, may have been out of the refrigerator for a while, and may have started to oxidize and ferment, which could upset your tummy. ***It should be fine for cooking, but not for raw soup. Make life interesting. Experiment to your heart's delight.***

Obviously, this does not represent the whole diet (at this stage). Treat it like part of your diet (the vegetable part). Keep to your usual way of preparing your food if you prefer, even if only for the time being. Get used to the new regime slowly. Instead of cooking your vegetables, try and eat them raw as described above. Do something you probably have never done before, combine them with fruit for taste (a salad). Be completely unconventional and add some vegetables to the fruit or visa-versa. There is no hard and fast rule. Use your imagination, become liberated. Why stick with convention?

A delicious salad dressing can be prepared by putting fruit together with natural flavouring in a blender, instead of using the commercial products with artificial ingredients.

Sprouts can easily be grown at home. All that is needed are four or five different kind of seeds, or as many as you like. The more the better.

Be bold, experiment, find different ingredients, as big a variety as possible. Try seeds like dark Lentils, dark Chickpeas, Moong beans, Fenugreek; anything you can think of that will sprout. Always keep to the dark colours. I eat sprouts almost every day of the week. What you do not eat raw, stir fry very lightly in, for instance, an omelette. You want to cook them as briefly as possible.

They are delicious with cheese sandwiches, in omelettes, or egg cakes. Fry the sprouts, break an egg over them and cook to serve as a filling in a sandwich. I would say that the most important ingredient in my entire diet after fruit is sprouts. They are so high in nutritional value and downright delicious. You don't have to stop at mere sprouts, allow them to reach small plant size, and "eat them, roots and all." They still remain the most nutritional food one could find. For salads, you may have to crop the roots which may be a little rough, or add them to your soup recipe. Good nutrition demands that sprouts should always be one of your first choices after fruit.

In a sunny spot in my apartment, I decided to experiment with growing tomatoes the hydroponic way. With a single plant, I eventually had many huge tomatoes. This made the neighbours very happy and they could not understand why I stopped growing them. The reason: I had so many tomatoes from one single plant that it eventually consumed too much living space.

How to get started growing sprouts? Begin on Friday evening (depending on the weather, summer or winter), put seeds in several 250 mill glass containers (cup). Quantities depend on the demand. Start with a small quantity the first time round, for the bigger seeds no more than one centimeter. Half fill the containers with water. Leave for 24hrs, pour off the water, rinse thoroughly, then lay the containers on their sides. It is important that they drain thoroughly. Raise the closed end a little.

Rinse the sprouts morning and evening until all have been consumed. It is important not to leave them standing in water once they have started sprouting They are vulnerable at this stage and could become very soft and can go off quickly. They should rather be consigned to the rubbish bin and not be eaten. Check for dead seeds after two to three days as they will ferment and upset the tummy. The shells of the Moong beans can be removed after one day in water by gently rubbing them against each other to loosen inside the cup, then leave to shed the shells on their own

Sounds like a mouthful, not really. By Monday evening your first harvest can be reaped and should last until Wednesday. To ensure the sprouts are young and fresh, start a fresh batch on Monday to be ready by Thursday. This routine can vary slightly between winter and summer. Quantities will have to be worked out according to demand. Should you arrange to sprout only once per week, by Wednesday remove all the husks. By Thursday or Friday, some of the sprouts may be a little too mature to be pleasant tasting. Chop them up and use them in your cooked dishes or soup. At this stage all the nutrients are present and the plant is at its best nutrition-wise. It can be compared with an infant animal, where the mother's milk is highly nutritious the first few weeks after birth to feed the young animal when it needs all the help it can get to start its new life successfully.

Include the sprouts in as many dishes as possible. The young ones are very tasty on their own or mixed with herbs or anything natural. Use your imagination, it does not take much effort.

It is very important not to overdo the blending. Stick to the suggestion mentioned above. It should not take more than a few seconds. The texture should still be a little coarse, to allow for some chewing which will ensure the mixture is well mixed with saliva. Before swallowing, move the mixture around in the mouth. Remember saliva is a digestive juice and the mouth is where the digestive process begins.

Sometimes I vary my evening meals with a large fruit and vegetable salad. Then you can use vegetables that are not suitable for a Smoothie. More often than not, it is more fruit than vegetables.

Being a vegetarian, I enjoy a vegetarian patty, just thawed and then eaten together with some grated and spiced beetroot, or any way you prefer, finishing my meal with dates, together with coconut (sweet tooth) or perhaps one single square of chocolate (kept in the refrigerator). This may seem a bit mean. Try it for yourself. Allow the chocolate to dissolve in your mouth. This can take some time and has the same effect as actively eating a lot more chocolate, fewer sugar calories, and the rest. *It is advisable to finish the meal with one, two or more slices of whole wheat bread to prevent constipation.*

Please do not destroy the whole exercise by adding large dollops of salad dressing indiscriminately. These are usually laden with sugar and salt, in my opinion, two commodities that should not be legally sold to the public without a danger warning on the packaging. The havoc these two evils wreak on health everywhere are legion. More on that in the chapter on sugar and salt. There are many recipes available, made up of natural ingredients like spices, mild vinegar, and many more. Go easy on the vinegar (allow the vinegar to drain off). It can be harsh and give rise to an imbalance in the metabolism. Yes, I know the body can handle it, but there is always the accumulated effect that should be taken into consideration when eaten often. Vinegar is an acid and should be taken in small quantities only.

Instead of a salad, I often simply dice the ingredients, pile them on a plate, and enjoy a delicious meal in front of the television. Dice an orange, apple, green beans, four different sprouts, small tomato, a slice of green pepper, parsley, small carrot and a small pear. Alternatively, an apple, large orange or slice of papaya, banana, small carrot, a small tomato and green pepper, whatever takes your fancy.

I should mention something about breakfast, the most important meal of the day. As it is so important, let's consider what goes into a super nutritious breakfast.

The easiest way to accomplish this would be to peep at what goes into my breakfast bowl. After my customary selection of delicious fruit, rolled oats only, not the kind touched by man's ingenuity to make it easy to prepare, instant, superfast, whatever. The best way to eat oats is to eat it raw. Sound ridiculous? Not really (100% nutrition). One small spoonful put through a grinder, together with one spoonful sunflower and linseeds – essential that the seeds are broken down in a grinder else they simply pass through the system – a medium size spoon soya powder, one large spoonful fine coconut (powerful protein), one spoon honey (to taste) dissolved in a little water, and lastly a very important ingredient, a large handful of bran flakes. Add whatever finds your fancy, as long as it is natural and nutritional, for instance a few spoons full of Muesli for taste.

Uncooked oats provide 100% nutrition and have been recognized as the best food for breakfast. The oats swell to several times its original size inside your stomach. That ensures bulk for long time sustenance.

If this breakfast can keep me climbing mountains until lunch time, I think it can do the same for you whatever occupies your day. Please do not think it too big or too much. It is absolutely non-fattening and has all the ingredients in the mix that are necessary for a highly nutritious healthy diet. Ladies can cut down on the quantities, but not on the ingredients.

Lunch time is when I consume my carbohydrates. Usually either rice with some olive oil, or four-grain soup which I cook like a stew or some whole wheat pasta. There are many varieties of carbohydrates as long as it is whole food. Unfortunately, they can only be consumed after being cooked

The mind plays a big role as to whether you will or will not accept a different diet. It is a powerful weapon. Remember you are in charge, your mind will accept any change you demand. When, after a while, it has accepted the change it is usually permanent. Approach it with an open mind, give yourself a chance try and enjoy the taste which will not be difficult. It is all delicious food.

Some people are so set in their ways it is difficult to change to a new way of eating. To them, it seems like a huge adventure. Well, be adventurous, you only live once.

If you are strapped for cash, there is no cheaper way to eat. If you had to buy peanuts for the same amount of money, the quantity would be considerably smaller. No amount of money can buy food with the same value in nutrition in a conventional way of eating, no matter how much money you want to spend.

Consider the benefits derived from a hugely improved lifestyle due to the increased energy supply.

Protein and enough of it, is a dire necessity in the diet. Where protein can arguably be considered to be superior to other nutrients is the fact that the building blocks, the cell, consist mainly of protein to make it possible for the other nutrients in the cell to perform their allotted functions up to the required standard. When the cells run short of protein to be able to keep functioning, water comes to the rescue. Water is a substitute, and like in most substitutes, more so in the body where it is not possible to supplant a nutrient as important as protein with something entirely different, performance must suffer.

Water which can't do the job adequately is less dense. Consequently, there has to be much more water than there would have been protein. Water is much heavier and bulkier, hence the person starts gaining weight, which is a very common problem and the average person is none the wiser why this is happening. *That is the reason why protein makes up the bulk of the ingredients in most weight-control products, vegetable or soya protein.*

Do not revert to using water tablets, or any other tablets for that matter. That is an unnatural and unhealthy way to try and achieve your goals. It is easy to pop a pill. The action is drastic to produce instant success, but how beneficial is this instant success to the benefit of long-term good health? Elvis Presley is a well-known name. At the tender age of forty-seven, he said goodbye to us leaving a huge void (his following was probably bigger than any other idol at the time). It all started with one, what may have been considered an innocent pill (for different reasons but it still remains an unnatural commodity, something alien to the metabolism), and then escalates out of control. Artificial chemicals (tablets) do not mix with and can't sub-plant the natural chemicals in the body.

If something is not natural, it is a good practice to always view such a product with suspicion. A name that made startlingly unpleasant news even more recently is that of Michael Jackson.

They were both healthy young men before they started taking pills for reasons that could have been satisfied in a more natural way. If at the moment you are still comparatively young and you should live to the age of sixty, or even older, you would not want to be in a situation where life is nothing more than purgatory, with a body that has become dysfunctional. That is not the time of your life to become a regular visitor to your doctor.

Think of the cost with runaway inflation on the medical front. The battles may be something you just could not handle. Remember *"old age is not for sissies."* There is a reason for this saying and it is true. Do your best to make things as easy as possible for yourself during those years. Always try and keep to the natural way when treating any deviation that occurs in the body. Most of the time it is far cheaper than artificial remedies. After all, your body is a natural creation and designed to respond to natural stimuli.

Vegetarians often have a psychological problem with protein. When the word protein is mentioned, it is automatically associated with meat. As meat is a no-no with vegetarians, a great substitute is usually preferred. Delicious dishes can be prepared with soya products that have been created with great care to deliver an up-to-standard ingredient for a healthy meal. Simply to view protein as overrated when the importance of health is taken into account is, to say the least, short-sighted.

A note of warning, you will find many varied opinions from outside on suggestions offered in this writing. Think carefully when you consider them. Not that I will ever claim that the opinions offered here are the only correct ones, but they are at least based on **common sense regarding natural nutrition.** After all, we are dealing with a very basic natural body with a basic natural metabolism.

There are, for instance, some opinions that soya is not altogether what it is made out to be. I personally have been taking soya protein for decades and have only positive results to show for it. At the same time, I am personally acquainted with a vegetarian who has different beliefs about protein. Unfortunately, she cannot back her beliefs with positive results. Just allow me to say that most objections are petty.

Be careful of irresponsible writings on health and related matters in magazines. I reiterate: stick to as close a relationship as possible with nature and natural foods when making a decision as to what to consume to enhance the state of or remain in good health. Nature never makes a mistake. We are the culprits when we lack the will to take proper care of our bodies to mistakenly take the easy way out. Life is precious and good health even more so.

It is possible that convictions, of which many of us are not aware, are the motivating factors behind the cause for confusion. Controversies have always found fertile ground where, due to a lack of interest, no personal research was done. Common sense should be the sensible way to go, and there will always be a difference of opinion. Whatever the argument, try and give the natural factor preference where the state of your future health is concerned.

To cut down on protein without giving it serious thought, perhaps through conviction, or simply ignorance, and then unwittingly avoiding this very necessary nutrient is a dangerous practice.

A word of warning: Do not listen to unsound advice obtained from dubious sources or hearsay, especially when health is on center stage. Musical chairs can be great fun, but leave that to less serious subjects. Get reliable information from reputable sources before making a serious decision. Another source of dubious information is the often heard "they say." One day I may just be so fortunate as to meet one of these very intelligent sources of wisdom who seems to be an all-wise lexicon on legs. A quality life can be had only by following good advice obtained from reputable sources.

The skin, the biggest organ in the body, is a prolific user of protein and when the skin is deprived of protein it becomes vulnerable, damages easily and ages prematurely, an anti-climax.

Vegetarians, when they go about things the right way, usually look much younger than consumers of meat products. It goes without saying that it is essential that protein is part of food intake every day and should not be regarded as less important than any other, rather as one of the most important parts of your nutritional intake.

The importance of protein cannot be over-emphasized and an adequate amount of protein consumption is very important. Let the mind wander from the smallest cell, which as stated earlier, consists mostly of protein (the most important building material ingredient), to the tissues and organs. They all need adequate amounts of protein. It will become apparent why protein is so important when the years start catching up with us and age begins to show by the appearance of skin that has been neglected, perhaps not willfully but through ignorance. (All the pulses and sprouts in the recipes above contain protein).

My personal choice of protein is soya, then extracts from milk as I am not partial to milk. The human race is the only creature that continues to take milk after being weaned. Using a product as strong and as powerful as milk can actually become destructive towards calcium, among others in the body. More is mentioned on milk elsewhere.

Is it possible to reverse an appearance that has aged prematurely on account of lack of proper nutrition? To an extent it is possible, by eating a lot more vegetable protein as well as following a more holistic diet for the recovery of the cells, and taking a somewhat larger than usual dose of vitamin A and D. These capsules are readily available, plus the extra protein are primarily for the benefit of the skin.

For the skeptics on vegetarian dishes and way of life, allow me to mention the difference I experienced when I first became a vegetarian. We have in the country where I live a national dish called, "Baboti." This must rank as one of the all-time favourites. The main ingredient is minced beef. At the time I had a friend who was an accomplished cook. She substituted the beef with soya mince. If anyone had told me beforehand that this particular dish could taste even better than the one made in the traditional way, I would have been skeptical.

After forty years of living on vegetarian food, I have learned that it is anything but boring and does not consist only of lettuce leaves and carrots. When cooking with meat the whole meal is usually built around the meat. Believe it or not, that leaves the cook with less latitude than would be the case with vegetarian dishes. There is no anchor around which vegetarian food is planned, so you have a wider scope to allow your imagination free reign. What I also discovered is that vegetarian dishes are a whole lot tastier than dishes prepared with meat being the center of attraction, not even mentioning the advantage on health it holds.

Any major change in life is predominantly a matter for the mind. When the mind is convinced of the overwhelming benefits compared to the other, the changeover is so much easier. The mind accepts it and then it is a fait accompli.

One often hears of some stimulant recommended to enhance performance of some sorts. To a certain extent that may be true, but there is no stimulant that can outperform a healthy nutrition-reared body where all the organs, muscles, and other body components are fed on first-class nutrition.

Perpetual motion does not exist. Wherever there is growth or motion, there has to be fuel to perform the necessary action. The quality of the fuel determines the level of performance, and the body is no different.

Consider the difference over a period of a lifetime between eating healthy food as described above, compared to consuming what I prefer to call dead food (cooked to death).

Allow me to mention one disease that is a frightening condition to have to contend with at an old age when it tends to strike: Osteoporosis (weakening of the bones in the body). Read more about this terrible condition in the chapter on exercises.

You often hear: This or that causes cancer. We don't know, but what is known is that good nutrition in a strong body can fight off cancer more successfully than a weak poorly nourished one.

Chapter 4

SUGAR / SALT

When I drive through the vast stretches of land devoted to the production of sugar cane, I never fail to wonder how so much land can be wasted on a commodity such as sugar. Apart from the enormous profits (billions) the moguls earn from it, there is very little good one can say for sugar. Apart from the fact that it supplies work to millions of people, I cannot think of a single plus mark one can award sugar. It is a commodity the world can easily do without completely. Considering the amount of damage done to the health of a large part of the population by the amount of sugar they consume, the product should be handled in a much more circumspect manner. There are so many ways one can satisfy the palate's craving for sweetness.

While flitting through the TV programs, one concerning diabetes caught my eye. It featured a presenter walking down the passage in a supermarket where thousands of products were displayed and she stated that it is impossible for the supermarkets to deny that they offer *starter kits for diabetes. She proceeded to physically demonstrate, using quantities stated on the packaging, how much sugar the average person consumes and she was especially perturbed at the amount children ingest.*

The body as a whole is simply not designed to cope with more than just a small amount. The detrimental after-effects of more than that is horrendous. The devastation that sugar wreaks all over the world on populations is of epidemic proportions. Diabetes vies for the number one spot when it comes to the cause of death. The number two spot will surely go to the effects obesity has on the body.

Perhaps thus far you have had luck on your side, for you have missed the dreaded disease, diabetes. It is commonly believed that when babies are overfed on an already poor diet together with sugar, the cells in the body become "fat" cells, for want of a better word, which grow together with the person, and it is very difficult for those people to control their weight upon reaching adulthood.

The less commonly known truth is that sugar is an unwelcome visitor to the body. The body is not designed to handle the oversupply of refined sugar. The body is designed to handle only natural sugar. More than just a small amount of refined ingested sugar causes mayhem in the body. The poor pancreas does its best to neutralize the situation, but eventually after the continuous abuse it is overwhelmed and the consequences for the owner of the body, to say the least, are dire, robbed of a life that could have been full of fun.

Should the situation not be beyond redemption, the noble hero, the holistic way of life, can come to the rescue so that not a perfect life, but a much improved one is still possible.

Together with salt and white flour, the three are known as the silent killers. At first, they cause people to become addicted to the effects they have on a person's metabolism. From then on it is a nasty ride to enormous suffering and an early death for a large percentage of the people who have become addicted to sugar and can't say no to the unnatural sweet taste. To die from the effects of diabetes is an awful and long road to travel that goes through many different stages, unfortunately, all of them representing tremendous suffering.

There are several different categories of diabetes. Sugar is not the only cause of diabetes, but the main contributor to a sad scenario, often in combination with other unhealthy eating habits like white flour.

The nerve system is the first to suffer. The nerve system touches not only every organ but every part right to the tiniest of cells, even every hair follicle. The whole body suffers. The first organs to feel the effects of devastation are the eyes, then the feet. Amputation of toes, feet and legs are not uncommon.

Even should you be so fortunate that fate will not be so cruel to you, the feet become so badly affected that it becomes an arduous task simply to walk. What a curtailment on movement and physical freedom. Are these warning signs not reason enough to reconsider your eating habits?

By now it is quite some time since the body started to protest against the treatment being meted out to it, not recognizing the reason for the lack of vitality and simply not feeling well. It may well be too late. A little knowledge on the noble subject, the holistic way of life, would have made all the difference. During the early stages of most diseases, holistic treatment can prevent enormous suffering and the rest of the person's life could still be lived to a reasonably happy conclusion. Unfortunately for diabetics, there is no going back, although life could be made a lot more comfortable if a holistic way of life were adopted from then on.

Once the problem has reached an advanced stage, the dreaded injections of Insulin several times per day begins. When the situation has reached this stage, the physical deterioration is irreversible and the suffering can last for several years. The time to start with a healthy holistic way of life is when we are children. Naturally, we do not have any say in the matter.

It is the responsibility of the parents to see to it that we do not follow the dreadful path so many folks do. *No doubt many parents do know that it is not to their children's benefit to eat these awful creations that are designed to appeal to the senses rather than good common sense.*

Sometimes, parents, being parents, find it hard to say no, knowing full well what they are doing is not right. They think "only this once" or "it's only a little," but unfortunately that is where good discipline falls flat and a bad habit is born. Sugar is an addictive substance, as has been explained before. The nerve system is where the problem will manifest itself. Every cell in the body is connected to the nerve system, and consequently the whole body will be adversely affected. It will be hard to convince me that the combination of too much sugar and poor nutrition is not the forerunner of children being administered the dreadful drug called **Ritalin** that has a calming effect on the child's nerve system.

The long-term effect of this drug is not always understood or recognized, especially on a brain that has not yet reached maturity. Later the person may develop some other problem, not realizing that the drug used, perhaps a long time ago, is responsible for the new problem. It stands to reason that any drug that has been designed to interfere with the workings of a delicate young organ, such as the brain when it was still in developmental stage, considered to be a normal creation without any diagnosed defects, can't be to the good of that organ or the nerves. This drug can be responsible for certain strange behaviour patterns manifesting only much later, which is often quite obvious to the more enlightened person, not so the parents who did not notice the gradual change in behaviour.

Chain reactions of this kind are often not recognized and can remain dormant for many years before manifesting behavioral symptoms, without their origin being realized. The brain is very different to any other organ and should be treated with respect, and a lot more circumspection. Being a very delicate organ, it needs good nutrition to stay healthy. What is good nutrition for the brain? There is no single answer to that question. The body is a natural creation, of which the brain is a part. It needs many different nutritional components found only in natural foods.

Imagine shaping and molding a child's psychological future with that kind of handicap to cope with, as well as the stress that goes with raising children. Granted, parents with all kinds of domestic problems are sometimes at a point where they do not know which way to turn. My heart bleeds for them, but don't make life even more difficult for yourself by feeding the child something that will affect his nerve system and eventually may lead to psychological problems, and make it more difficult for you to handle the already strained situation.

Do not allow your child to become addicted to sugar. The consequences will be a lot harder to cope with than the effort to make them understand that it is for their own benefit to be denied those tantalizing tidbits that were created with profits in mind. Nature has provided us with many wonderful foods to satisfy the craving for sweets and you can eat to your heart's delight. What comes to mind? Fruit, dried fruit, dates, etc. It does not take long for the brain to accept the new habit and then all is plain sailing, the old tastes forgotten.

The scenario described above is only one of many instances where individuals have never experienced the wholesome and wonderful existence that is to be found with a natural way of living. *How often parents, without being any the wiser, were responsible for some horrendous conditions, such as biological, physiological, emotional, and even nerve warfare within their child or children.* With a little foresight and knowledge, it could have been so different. Life is meant to be simple. We tend to make it complicated by looking for answers that are staring us in the face, ignoring them for being too simple. Prevention is not only better than cure, it is the only way.

Make it a rule in your life to always try and follow the natural route. Our bodies are, after all, natural creations and to introduce too many unnatural commodities and habits is not a good idea. The two together do not make good bedfellows.

As mentioned before, there are several different types of diabetes, and only a small percentage are not caused by poor nutrition. It could have been so very different had these persons taken heed of warnings such as these writings and many other tell-tale signs, and so avoid heartache and hardship. Sad to say, these warnings are so often ignored even though they are usually not issued with sensation in mind nor for profit, but to explain a better lifestyle, hence a world with less suffering. Often the motivation comes from first-hand experiences, such as seeing a loved one suffer.

The relationship between sugar and energy supply is often misunderstood. It is true that sugar creates an energy boost. Unfortunately, it is not sustainable for long. What happens is, the ingested sugar, which is highly toxic to the body (in other words it is really a poison), has to be neutralized as soon as possible. The pancreas releases insulin to do the job. It is the insulin which is there to neutralize the effect of the sugar that creates the sudden boost of energy that is of short duration on account of the contaminated insulin being immediately absorbed by the body into the digestive system after the job has been done.

For a long and sustainable energy supply, one needs the assistance of complex carbohydrates which are designed for sustainable energy supply. These are foods like honey, fruit, rice, maize, and all the whole grain foods like bread and some pasta products. They are all natural wholesome products, provided they have not yet been contaminated by man's evil genius.

For a long and sustainable supply of energy, for instance during a sporting event, it is important to go on to what is known as "carbo loading," eating copious amounts of carbohydrates for several days prior to the event. The body stores the chemicals which are released as required. This point is slightly controversial as to its effectiveness, like so many holistic ideas denigrated by unenlightened persons. Trying it can do no harm and may very well be beneficial.

Honey is a natural sustaining substance for a long lasting energy supply. Honey is pre-digested food and is immediately absorbed directly into the bloodstream through this wonder of nature, the membrane in the mouth, particularly under the tongue, it is designed to absorb the honey and pass it on directly into the blood stream.

Do not swallow the honey immediately, swirl it around in your mouth for maximum effect. Together with oxygen, they make a formidable team to make sure the muscles receive the necessary fuel to do the job you require them to do properly. For this particular purpose, honey is a powerful substance and it is advisable to dilute it with an equal or more quantity of water. This is the ideal mix and should be sipped and not taken by the mouthful, to create energy for anybody who indulges in strenuous sport such as long distance running.

SALT is a partner in crime. The scenario is the same although it causes a very different disease, affecting the body in a totally different but equally disastrous way.

Being equally insidious, the craving for salt begins in a small way. Perhaps just developing a liking for the taste or the preposterous idea that everything the body ingests needs a lot of salt. Very little salt should be taken. Natural salt is already provided in the food we eat. Another misguided reason is to show off – something I have witnessed first-hand when someone passes an innocent friendly warning concerning the use of too much salt to someone who should know better. The ego suffers and it could be the beginning of long-term suffering. *It is erroneous to blame water for the extra weight. It is the excess salt that causes the retention of water to neutralise the dangerous effect the salt would otherwise have on the body.*

The first negative effect is usually weight-gain, and it is easy to understand why. Salt, or sodium chloride as it is known scientifically, is such a drastic chemical which does not assimilate with the metabolism. The body certainly does not need it in excess and can only tolerate it in very small quantities for a limited period of time. The body has no defense against the onslaught, other than the natural way and that is to dilute the effects of salt with water. Sodium in small quantities is essential for good health and is available in other foods.

The normal reaction after eating something salty is to drink water. In this instance, where there is a continuous oversupply of salt, the body stores the water in order to cope with the after-effects, resulting in water retention to neutralize the harmful effects of salt. Water is a heavy commodity, consequently the person suffers weight gain.

The body is not designed to handle the effects of too much salt. The blood density increases and it is in the blood stream where the first negative symptoms are noticed. Higher blood pressure than normal is experienced. This harmful condition usually escalates into headaches. From there on, one of several different calamities can follow – blood clots forming then stroke, or heart attack, is the end result.

The brain needs a constant supply of oxygen to function. The slightest interruption of the supply by a blood clot can be catastrophic. I think all of us have seen the effects on a person who has suffered a stroke. It usually affects only one side of the body, a sad sight indeed.

Once again, allow me to say that not all strokes are salt induced. There are several different causes, but salt remains by a large margin the main culprit and one that could easily have been avoided. There is nothing good to be said about the use of too much salt. If I may quote my own experience as an example, I have not had salt in my household for decades. The only salt I consume is in the occasional pre-prepared product, like a vegetarian patty, or the fact that I live at the coast where sea air is usually saturated with salt. The body requires sodium in minute quantities, and the salt I ingest in this way is more than enough to fill the need. Use salt sparingly to fill the need for sodium. Go easy on the intake of salt.

The old wives tale that one needs salt or salt tablets to avoid cramps remains just that, an old wives tale.

I live in a subtropical to tropical climate, am an outdoors person, climbing mountains in the hot African sun which has been a passion all my life. I have not had a single negative effect from the heat or the sun, certainly no cramps. Many times, though, I had to assist where people have suffered the effects of excessive heat. Could it be that excessive use of salt left the victim more vulnerable and has to bear some responsibility?

The craving for salt is an acquired taste. Unfortunately, children are fed salt almost from birth. Only when the dreadful habit has been kicked out of existence, can one appreciate how delicious vegetables and many other foods are where the taste has not been spoiled by the use of salt.

Food cooked in waterless cookware, where there is none or very little water present, means absolutely no salt or condiments are needed. In fact, condiments would hide the delicious natural taste of freshly cooked vegetables. Try it, the taste will prove to be a revelation. It must be one of the easiest acquired tastes. There is no water present to wash the natural salts, sugars, and nutrients out of the food. Should you want to cook your food, then this is the way to do it.

Allow me to dispel a myth that one needs to buy expensive waterless cookware. All that is needed is for the cookware to have a thick aluminum or copper base, together with a reasonably well fitting lid. That, one can say with confidence due to modern day engineering techniques, comes standard.

After rinsing the vegetables, add no more than a spoonful of water. Start on medium heat and when the vapours start to escape from the lid, turn the heat down to an absolute minimum. The nutrition remains intact. **What a tremendous improvement over the traditional way of cooking.**

The argument for sodium in the diet certainly has some merit. The amount of sodium needed for optimum health, like most forms of nutrition, is minute. Enough sodium can be had via the regular healthy food eating routine, a multivitamin or even the occasional pre-prepared food or occasional snack the holistic way of life enthusiast will ingest during the normal course of the day. A holistic way of life does not make for a boring existence. It is what is done on a regular basis that matters.

Should you be a victim of high blood pressure and are on medication, a good idea would be to have the blood pressure tested weekly (some pharmacies do that as a free service to pensioners). When the pressure returns back to normal, stop taking the medicine.

The lack of sodium in the body can manifest itself with a slight feeling of light-headedness and a dry sensation on the lips. The solution to the problem may be quite simple. Dissolve a teaspoon tip of salt in hot water and drink it. Should the symptom persist, seek medical advice.

The third enemy of our precious good health is **white flour**. Because I am so dead against eating anything made from white flour, I cringe every time I see a person putting that dreadful stuff into their mouth. Why am I so vehemently against white flour?

The way flour, yes wonderful flour, the staff of life, has been brutalized and then presented as food that is supposed to be a nutritional creation designed to feed the body, is now sterile, it resembles, and is equally as nutritious as a wad of cotton wool. *All the nutritional material has been removed and is used to manufacture other products such as, for instance, vitamins (extra profit, at what cost to the unsuspecting public). The variety and volume of food, if one can call it food, that is made from white flour is astonishing. (Stop for a moment and realise the amount of food made from sterile white flour). Why should this be so one may ask? To earn more revenue, subsequently more profits,* I am sure is the answer. Advertising is incredibly powerful. Why care about the welfare of the nation if you can earn more money and get away with it. On the other hand, the nation is equally to blame. It is so easy, and absolutely a necessity, that the nation becomes educated about good nutrition. Good nutrition is not a luxury, and to acquire it is just simple common sense. The level of gullibility that leads to ignorance is mind-blowing.

The equally diabolical advertising industry, together with manufacturers, have only one thing in mind and that is profit. It is an industry that is psychologically highly-developed to dupe the consumer into believing almost anything. Blatant lying is not only accepted, it has become almost compulsory to lie, in this instance without interference by the authorities. Unfortunately, it is so insidiously done that the average person who is not sufficiently informed to recognize such instances when they do occur, is the one who suffers.

I was involved with the advertising industry for many years, but thankfully not anymore. To mention just one example: A new washing powder is introduced to the public. The total cost of setting up the plant would be a certain amount which will be minute compared to the amount budgeted for advertising, possibly as little as one-tenth of the total budget, and the balance which is negligible in comparison to getting the plant up and running would account for the rest of the expenditure. This single product will eventually be turned into a multimillion dollar venture. It is suggested to be the end all and be all of soap powders, and the reasons why it is the best ever are beamed to tens of millions out there. If only one million packets are sold initially a lot of revenue is generated, and the product is no different to any other, bar perhaps the smell.

Does advertising pay? You bet it does. This exercise can still be tolerated when it concerns material matters, but please leave the food we ingest into our precious bodies alone. ***The combination of sugar and white flour must surely be a major cause of diabetes.***

Chapter 5

THE HEART

Our greatest friend, the heart, is one of the few machines in existence capable of perpetual motion, followed closely by the brain and the lungs, and they are all found in one unit, that miraculous entity, the body. They do need nutrition for maintenance, but no fuel or any other form of propulsion is needed to drive these organs. The heart is also the most important driving force in the body. Short of a heart transplant, all else can fail to a certain extent and life can still be sustained, but should the heart stop functioning everything stops and the end of life will have been reached. Could this be why so much mythology flows from the heart? The beginning of life, the end of life, and so much in between, our heart, the seat of all emotion.

It is essential that the heart gets all the support that is humanly possible to ensure an enjoyable lifestyle and a lot more, when sport or any other activity demands more than the heart can deliver, no matter how big the demand.

In one respect the heart is just like any other muscle in the body, the harder it works the stronger it becomes. When one thinks of the enormous demand made by athletes practicing extreme sport on the heart (and the body), one can be forgiven for thinking that its power to deliver is unlimited. That is true, provided the care is adequate and we supply the necessary exercise and nutrition – the fuel and building material. Should we fail to take adequate care by not feeding the body tissue the necessary nutrients, we do pay a price for being negligent and this becomes obvious when our bodies do not live up to expectations by starting to break down long before we expect it to, or become ill when they really should not.

Bar accidents, birth defects, contagious diseases and the like, the average human body is designed to last for a very long time, well into old age without getting sick, provided the necessary hygienic conditions inside the body exist and care and maintenance are as natural as possible. Wild animals do not get sick provided they never come into contact with humans. They are born healthy, live their lives under extreme conditions such as snow, rain, and heat, and die at an old age.

We humans are the privileged part of creation, same design but with more privileges than animals, so why do we become ill so often? Consider the state of health generally worldwide. It is frightening. When we neglect to care for our most precious possession, the body, by not supplying it with the necessary nutrition or performing the necessary exercise to build strength and stamina so that we can live a life that is prosperous, exciting and full of fun, and take part in any sport to our liking and ability, we will not be able to perform all these wonderful feats.

We are not all gifted to the same extent in all aspects of life, and sport is no different. Try any sport until you find one that appeals to you. It is important that we play sport or at least take part in some activity that stretches our muscles, including the heart, until we feel the endorphins coursing through our arteries, veins, and muscles, a wonderful experience. Once hooked you will not want to stop.

Like everything worthwhile, the initial effort could be trying, but once you are reasonably fit the going gets easier and then the enjoyment starts. The enjoyment and benefits are enormous.

Then the quality of life really moves up a notch or two, with lots of energy and you feel like you can move mountains. The brain livens up, we make new friends, social life improves. and much more. It does not happen overnight, it takes time, and it is advisable to go slowly but do **persevere.** It is well worth the effort.

When we are unfit it is fairly hard work to get into shape but don't let that scare you, we always get out a lot more than we put into a fitness program. It is like a motor car traveling at a reasonable speed, it takes a lot less effort to maintain a constant speed, and playing sport is the same. You leisurely coast along and will not be able to wait to get back to doing what you so detested before and enjoy so much now. Allow me to clarify what I am saying. I climb the stairs of twenty-one floors regularly. To the uninitiated, this may sound like being equal to a small mountain. Not really, when I get to the top my breathing has increased marginally, my pulse rate increases by a mere ten beats per minute. I am no different to any other person. Exercise is part of my life. You can do the same and enjoy life so much more.

What has all this got to do with the heart? It is the engine that drives this marvellous train, the body, and makes all the fun possible. The heart, like all the muscles in the body, needs to be brought up to standard to be able to perform. Exercise is the most important aspect after nutrition to achieve this goal. In the case of beginners of any age, start slowly.

At first, walk once around the block (start with a small one). Keep that up for four or five days, and if you feel like doing it twice the first time, by all means, go for it. The following week double the effort. Keep up the progress for perhaps a month, and then it is time to join a walk/run club. Many sport-loving people began in this way. Before long you will be joining the ranks of the adrenalin junkies.

An example to show what is possible if we don't all have the desire to achieve such high ideals: an acquaintance started her running career at age sixty-four. During the next decade she completed several long distance events, including a marathon, and at age seventy took part in the senior world championships and was eventually the proud owner of a few world records. Now in her mid-eighties, she is still pounding the roads. Is that something to be proud of or what? No boredom when she is around. We are not all the same. Should you be of a more sedentary persuasion, which is by far the largest group, no problem, you more than likely enjoy watching television. Make a very small change to your pastime and acquire an exercise bicycle; what is known as a going-nowhere bike.

At entry level, they come at a very reasonable price, and that is all you need, something cheap and simple. Sit on your bike in front of the television set while watching your favourite soapy, set the resistance at the lowest level or do not set the resistance at all, just allow your legs go around for as long as it suits you. You are getting exercise, and from there you progress at your own pace. Exercise is vitally important for good health. You will always be rewarded by receiving more than you put into the effort you make.

One important aspect about the heart – the tissue is very different to the rest of the body. Should one suffer an injury or it is severely neglected, it heals at a much slower pace, and sometimes it does not heal at all. Check with your physician before you start any sport that requires above a reasonable rate of activity It is important to look after one's heart with great care.

Two young friends come to mind, one in his thirties, great social life, overweight, smoking, big around the waist. The other in his early twenties, similar in lifestyle, except the latter did not drink or smoke. I never consciously tried to influence their way of life. Whenever we met, inevitably the subject of health and well-being came up for discussion. The story has a happy ending, the first stopped smoking and both became ardent exercise and fitness enthusiasts. Imagine how their lives changed.

Recently I met with the younger one and remarked on how well he looked. Even his hair looked so healthy it was difficult not to notice. His response took me by surprise. "I am following your advice; healthy lifestyle, eating sensibly, a moderate exercise routine, and not washing with soap, not even my hair. I haven't washed with soap for some time now."

A change such as this to any person's life is worth far more than money can buy. It all revolves around the condition of the heart, where it all begins. Look after it well and follow the advice found in the chapter on Nutrition and it will serve you selflessly and reward you handsomely for many years with lots of joy and happiness, well into old age.

While on the subject of nutrition: The most important vitamin for the heart is vitamin C. On account of the fact that it elasticises tissue, all tissue, it is of utmost importance to the heart muscles and arteries, which are of different tissue to the rest of the body. It keeps the arteries open, strong, supple, and in good condition. At least 300mg per day is the minimum requirement.

Another very important mineral to ensure your heart stays healthy and happy is potassium. No need to rush off and buy potassium nutrients, one banana per day will do the job admirably. It will prevent fibrillation and if the condition should occur, the same treatment will rectify the heart rhythm and in many instances, obviate the fitting of a pacemaker.

Chapter 6

BLOOD

It is almost impossible to talk about the heart and not mention blood. Let's put that right. The heart, arteries, veins or vascular system, plus the blood, makes up the transport system in the body. The blood moves the nutrition from the intestines where it was absorbed to the relevant organs, muscles, bones, tissue material, even the tiniest cells. Nothing is left out, no matter how small. Amazing, imagine a big fellow... hard to believe that it is nutrition that keeps him alive and healthy. All that his huge body needs to sustain itself comes in the form of nutrition so small you would not be able to see it with the naked eye.

This is the building material that feeds the cells that make up the skin on his small toe and is brought to that area by the blood, transported from the intestines where it was received, via the arteries. Is there anything more amazing anywhere on earth? It is not only man that is treated in this very special way. All related life forms are served in the same manner.

Just think how many different components comprise nutrition. As laymen, we would be guessing. When a person is not well, to determine what is ailing him, the first thing normally requested is a blood test to make it possible for the physician to make an accurate assessment. That gives us an idea how much nutrition, or the lack thereof, is present in the blood

The easiest way to rid yourself of a feeling of malaise after a spell of inactivity is to start moving, the more rapidly the better. The muscles require energy, the blood enriched with oxygen and nutrition obliges, and there is an instant feeling of well-being.

Vital signs such as the heartbeat, blood pressure, and breathing, are all to do with blood and the quality thereof. When the cleanliness of the inner body (the vascular system as well as the digestive system) is mentioned, it refers to the state of cleanliness of the blood. The cleaner the inner body, (in other words the blood), plus good nutrition, the more ideal are those signs that indicate the state of health and wellbeing the body enjoys at that particular moment.

When these measurements are taken, the body must be in a state of rest and relaxed for a few minutes. For example, the ideal blood pressure is 115/75. The ideal pulse rate varies, for the average none-sporting but healthy person, about 65, down to an extremely fit and healthy sports-conscience person, around 50 beats per minute. Should these figures increase by a reasonable margin, it does not mean your health is not as good as you would like it to be, but perhaps that you are only less fit than you would like to be or should be.

Top athletes, like cyclists or ironman competitors, are arguably the fittest athletes in the world and it is not uncommon for them to register a pulse rate of fewer than 50 beats per minute. I must stress, should your pulse rate be anywhere near as low as 50-60 and you class yourself as a nonsporting person, do see your regular physician as by now you would have realized that all is not well. Should the reading be any higher than the average of 70 please do not be alarmed until you have been assessed by either a medical or sporting professional. These are merely guidelines. Needless to say, one should have a general medical assessment at least once a year after the age of sixty.

After being assessed by a professional and found to be in a reasonable state of health, but not quite to your expectations, that would be a good time to make a start at following the advice given elsewhere and put things right by following a better diet and fitness regime to start enjoying life.

The blood includes oxygen that has already been converted to energy ready for use, and the blood must do the job of getting it to the muscles. Consequently, even the slightest movement will cause a pro-rata increase in the pulse rate. As the movement or exercise becomes more vigorous, the muscles need more fuel to operate.

As mentioned before, the body thrives on exercise, the harder it works the stronger and healthier it becomes and it will not be long before you will start enjoying the change of lifestyle. Think of body builders for instance, how hard they work, and the results they achieve. They are usually very happy people.

Speaking from experience, the joy and pleasure one gets from being fit can only become a reality by being there and doing it. This is not something one can explain. Joining the ranks of adrenalin junkies is a worthwhile pastime and is highly recommended.

We do not have to strive to be top athletes, just aim to be moderately fit and get the best out of life. The effort is so worthwhile. These are all the good points about blood. The small percentage that takes the trouble and makes an effort to be concerned about their health, are the ones that have discovered how incredibly joyful life can be.

The flip side of the coin is an entirely different story altogether. The biggest item that keeps the tills humming at hospitals is, of course, heart attacks, and most of the time the cause of this plague of our society is blood that is saturated with cholesterol. This condition is caused by sheer neglect and ignorance. Allow me to say before I am shot down in flames, I know there are victims (a small minority) who suffer the dreaded condition where the body produces an inordinate amount of cholesterol without being stimulated to do so, and they have my heartfelt sympathy. As for the rest, a good diet (that does not mean everybody must become vegetarians, just a little more good judgment) will make the world of difference. More on this point can be found elsewhere in chapters pertaining to this problem.

There is no truer saying than **you are as young as your arteries.** That also includes the quality of the blood, that valuable carrier of the cargo loaded with nutrients which are transported throughout the body nonstop twenty-four seven. Our bodies never sleep, only our minds do. Sleep provides the rest that builds stamina and produces the energy we need at the beginning of every new day. As the heart beats the blood is refreshed, replenished with all the nutrition the body, including the brain, needs to keep functioning properly. The blood that is so valuable deserves a little more consideration by providing it with better quality fuel to do its work

During times of injury, one should exercise as vigorously as possible, without causing more damage to the injured area. Blood is a healer, the more nutrition, in other words, the more blood the injured area receives the faster the recovery from the injury.

Our pets are often better looked after health-wise than we are. Most people go to great lengths to make sure their pets get the best nutrition available. They will not hesitate to deny them food that is detrimental to their health, yet they will eat with gay abandon what they surely know is not good for their own health. Not that I would like to see our pets treated with less care, but we should just make an effort to apply the same criteria to ourselves.

Chapter 7

ARTERIES

*E*ver heard *"You are only as healthy as your arteries?"*
*That's very true. Those of us who have witnessed open
heart surgery on television will remember what an
artery looks like after fifty or sixty years of hard work. It is
hard to believe that something so worn, so unhealthy
looking, managed to sustain life right up to that moment.
Dull in colour, anything but the healthy pink it should be, a
lifeless object which is really a tube, out of which the life has
been wrung by sheer negligence and an erroneous belief
that this is normal and par for the course that an all-wise
God has destined for them.*

Let's be honest and say it is sheer negligence or ignorance. Let's kick
this habit once and for all of believing that we have no responsibility
towards ourselves, our families, our loved ones, everybody who
depends on us for a living, the ones who look up to us for leadership,
guidance and moral support, in some cases perhaps even society itself.

To think that we do not have to educate ourselves in the basic
knowledge of how to maintain a responsible lifestyle is sheer self-
indulgences and ignorance. Enough attention is continuously drawn to
the subject of care and maintenance of one's body, and in particular the
vascular system that includes the heart.

The "victim" did not heed the warning to take the necessary interest
and effort in maintaining a healthier eating regime to make sure the
body receives the required nutrition to sustain a healthy lifestyle. It also

did not receive the necessary care in avoiding eating harmful, or too much food. It received no exercise, or not enough to make it strong enough to combat the battles of life. Remember the more exercise the body receives, the stronger and more robust does it become. Most important, though, a healthy diet should be the first priority.

What are neglected arteries? The walls of the artery have collapsed and lost their elasticity. Add to that, the fact that the artery walls were, without a doubt, lined with cholesterol. Consider how hard the heart had to labour, pumping blood to the rest of the body through clogged up canals in such poor condition. It does not bode well for the achievement of a long healthy life with energy in abundance. A quality of life, in general, boils down to healthy eating habits and exercise. It is very difficult to reconstitute any tissue like that of arteries at such an advanced stage of deterioration.

An effort can be made to bring about an improvement to the condition with the help of large doses of nutritional supplements (vitamins C and E). Hoping for an improvement? Certainly, you can. Expect it to return to prime condition? The answer is a definite no. It is, therefore, imperative that one starts while still in one's prime. Take responsibility for your own health to preserve the quality that is available, whatever stage in life you are at, and arrest the deterioration if need be. Should there be any doubt as to the quality of the arteries, have yourself tested and whatever the outcome, improvements to a better lifestyle (good nutrition) should be implemented without delay, the most important vitamin, same as for the heart, is Vitamin C, 300 mg per day.

We have not yet reached the stage where nirvana is a reality. We can live in a fool's paradise in a reckless fashion and hope for the best, or we can take the more realistic alternative route. Take hold of the measure of youth that is still left within you and make that last as long as possible. Whatever your age and physical condition, a vast improvement is possible.

Think for a moment and consider the difference. Your body is one thing in life that comes free, gratis, and for nothing. All we have to do is make the effort to maintain and service what we have. We go to great lengths to make sure our motor cars receives proper care, the correct oil in the engine, different oil for the gearbox and differential, all kinds of additives.

The argument is: if I don't take good care of my motor car it will cost a fortune in the end. Dear friend, the same attitude will cost you a whole lot more to put anything right in the body that went wrong, if at all possible.

Why be so careless with our own health? There is evidence all around us of people in a neglected state of health. Caring for our health and well-being is very, very rewarding, ensuring a healthy body that will supply endless happiness and enjoyment. Break the destructive habit of living only for the moment, eating and drinking what appeals to our debased culinary senses without considering the consequences. Remember there is no reason to deprive ourselves entirely of a delicious steak or any other red meat dish as long as we do so in moderation and good sense. *It is what we do and eat on a regular basis that matters, not what we do occasionally.*

Circulation is the operative word here, getting the individual nutrients where they are needed to keep the rivers, streams and creeks, the transport system of the body, clean and free of obstacles and rough surfaces and in good condition to make it easier for the heart to pump the nutrients where they are needed. When the quality of the circulatory process is impaired or interrupted, the building materials are not delivered on time, or are of poor quality, or perhaps not getting there at all, the superstructure will suffer and the quality of the arteries themselves and that of the entire body, will be below par, affecting health and living life at half throttle or even less.

Most people who fall into this category are much of the time well aware that life is not what it is, could, and should be, and out of sheer ignorance accept the situation and consequences as inevitable. To them, this is the way it was meant to be. A happy spirit can only live in a healthy body, mind, and soul.

To make sure all the nutritional requirements of the arteries are catered for, it is advisable for those on a regular meat diet to take a regular daily dose of Vitamin E (400 int. units) which will help keep the arteries clear of cholesterol, together with a dose of Vitamin C (300 mill. grams) to ensure the heart and artery tissue retain its elasticity. Please don't see this as a license to ignore good eating habits.

Poor circulation is caused by neglecting the body in general, mostly on account of not enough or no exercise.

The above mentioned are usually not obvious to the layman. The person will only gradually become aware that all is not well. The first signs of breakdown in functions of the circulatory system are aches and pains in the lower legs, beginning at around middle age. We have been inactive for some time now, maintaining a sedentary lifestyle, perhaps what we mistakenly call a good life. Developing some pains in the lower legs, thinking that it is par for the course, we do not pay much attention to the situation until it gets worse and it is time to see a doctor or some other professional. Prevention is better than cure and when conditions have reached this stage, one has already lost some elasticity in the arterial tissue that cannot be restored. Young people, look after your health, there is no second time around.

The human race is at a slight disadvantage because we walk upright. The heart has a huge mountain to climb on account of being situated high in the body. The workload is much heavier for the human heart than it is for other animals. It has to pump the blood all the way down to the feet, which is not so bad. The return journey is a different story altogether. Not only does it have to pump the blood down, it has to force blood back up to the top with the same movement. Unless the arteries and veins are in good shape it really is hard work.

When conditions mentioned above begin to form, the heart loses efficiency and the result is the beginning of poor circulation. It is fairly easy to detect this. The area just below the ankle on the inside of the foot should be clear. If there is what looks like a miniature roadmap developing, it is time to get involved in a much more vigorous activity than is the case at that moment. It will make the heart stronger, and will, therefore, be able to move the blood with less effort throughout the body, in the process increasing the blood flow and improving the circulation. Do not forget to improve your nutritional intake. The "roadmap" may not necessary disappear. It is dead and calcified spider veins which cannot be resurrected. Not a train smash.

If it is still in the beginning stages it will not affect life severely, in which case consider yourself lucky, you have been warned in time. The ones not so fortunate are those who ignored the warning and are moving on to the next stage in the line of development, or a better word to fit the situation would be a line of destruction. That would be blood clots forming. The situation has now developed into a serious condition, an indication conditions in the whole vascular system are not what they should be, and the traumatic prospect of having stents fitted to keep the arteries open could be a very real possibility.

Stents are relatively small compared to the rest of the system, and don't think that the problem has been solved. It will just as easy for the problem to repeat itself somewhere else.

The blood carrying the necessary nutrients is not getting through to where they are needed, consequently they cannot make repairs and perform the necessary maintenance work.

What is even more serious is the fact that oxygen can't get through to the heart muscles, with dire consequences. The tissue is slowly dying and in severe cases, where conditions have taken on serious proportions and have become quite obvious, is not a pleasant sight to see and evokes a feeling of pity. "If only" is a thought often expressed, but always too late. It could have been very different. You have either deprived yourself of a large chunk of life, or at best live a shortened life at half-throttle.

Bed sores are a tragic and very painful condition which is not always due to neglect. This condition arises when the heart cannot move the blood through the arteries fast enough due to inactivity, which is not always the fault of the person, or where poor circulation is responsible, which could be due to several different reasons. Massaging becomes the only way to keep the circulation moving to prevent bedsores from forming, which can only be done by another person who is not always available. This is where the good Samaritans (where available) step in to offer their time, free of charge, to bring relief to these poor hapless people. We can be truly grateful for these angels of mercy.

Just another reason for maintaining good quality arteries is that the blood will flow much more easily through clean well-maintained arteries. It may not prevent adverse conditions from setting in eventually, but at least will delay their appearance long enough to make a difference.

Once bedsores have made their appearance, massaging is not always possible. With older people, it becomes a whole lot more difficult. Naturally, circulation complications can appear all over the body. These are just two examples. Moral of the story: eat sensibly, keep exercising, keep active, and keep moving.

This sounds like a whole lot of hard work (usually for these unfortunate victims), but believe it or not, a changed lifestyle for the better is not tantamount to a sentence to hard labour. It can become addictive and that will prove to be a mind-blowing experience. It will prove to be an achievement, even though a small one, the hallmark of a happier life.

Chapter 8

LUNGS

Ever given those two marvelous and amazing pumps in your chest cavity more than a passing thought? Yet another case of perpetual motion, lungs doesn't need any fuel source or battery to drive them. They do pretty well by themselves, thank you very much. Not even man with his incredible ingenuity and the awesome cyber world at his disposal, can produce anything remotely like the lung to do the same work. There is the artificial lung available to surgeons in operating theatres, but it is easier to fit man into that machine than the other way around. The lungs never stop or miss a stroke, just keep going twenty-four seven, from the moment of birth until the end, seventy, eighty years later. Our body is indeed wonderfully made, but unfortunately so often taken for granted. It never receives so much as a thought or sympathy for the conditions we subject our lungs to that are within our power to change or improve, but blatantly abuse them, like smoking for instance.

The lungs are constructed of delicate sponge-like tissue, fine and minute veins, and arteries, small tubes, and what can almost be described as minute little tunnels. When one considers all this delicate construction, the demands made upon them are mindboggling. The litres of air that pass through them depending on the demands made by the different movements supplying the oxygen to be converted into energy, compels one to see the lungs in a different light altogether.

The main function of the lungs is to supply the body with an adequate volume of oxygen, to be processed into energy, which the blood distributes to every cell in the body. This happens at an incredibly fast rate. Imagine the amount of oxygen an athlete requires during a race or any sportsman that requires physical energy to perform.

How is it possible for any part of the body to be subjected to so much hard work and just keep on doing what it was designed to do without complaining? A quick answer would be exercise and nutrition, feeding fuel to those amazing little cells doing what they are designed to do, and so keeping the body not only healthy but making it stronger. The harder it works, the healthier and stronger it becomes, no wear and tear, just the opposite. It is not only the human race but many other creatures with similarly structured bodies, that possess lungs with this amazing ability to grow stronger with use, provided they are continuously supplied with an adequate amount of oxygen, which is a major part of nutrition.

How can we make life a little easier for the lungs so they can do their work better, make them healthier, and happier, apart from good nutrition? Definitely with exercise, and the most common, most natural and arguably still the best exercise is walking. Walking is a natural action and comes easily to the body. The variation is wide, starting from a leisurely stroll for sheer enjoyment and increasing the pace to fit the level of your requirements. There is no limit as to how far you can or want to push your ability, walking is always a winner.

Many people enjoy pushing themselves to the limit while walking, but most are quite happy to maintain a leisurely pace. There is nothing wrong with that attitude. Would it not be so much better to add a little competition and enjoy a whole lot more benefit. Simply become a walker with a more structured program, add a little planning to the process. Walk a little faster or a little further, and you will find it will be so much more interesting, a wonderful way of getting into the swing of things. You will be surprised at how soon you get bitten by the bug, and the beginning of an altogether new lifestyle.

The most important thing we can do apart from exercise to keep the lungs hale and hearty, and to make it easier for them to operate and perform the awesome task of keeping us alive, well, and in prime condition, is to assume a decent posture at all times. Sit and move in an upright position, back straight, shoulders square, and chest out. This stance will free the lungs, which do not have an awful lot of room to move and process enough energy for the body's needs, no matter what the requirements are. This action will also prevent the forward slump, a condition many people suffer from often because of psychological reasons. Among these are very tall people. Be proud to be tall, most people who are not would love to be taller.

The danger of this posture is that the lungs **cannot** expel **all** the stale air, which can be detrimental to health. Air is a living commodity and like all things live, when it dies it will eventually putrefy. The body has the capacity to rid itself of some of the putrefied air by way of waste management, but not entirely, which could lead to problems of a very serious nature.

As usual, the importance of direct nutrition must not be underestimated. The lungs have a very large surface area. If it were possible to open the lungs and spread each little follicle side by side, the area it covers would be enormous. This whole surface area is covered by the mucous membrane. This membrane, because of its size and complicated construction and vulnerability, requires an enormous amount of nutrition compared to the rest of the body. The main vitamin would be vitamin A in combination with several other vitamins, the same as all the other organs and parts of the body. Complicating matters by describing all the nutrition the lungs require to keep them happy is not the object of this book. That is information that can be had from various reliable sources like the internet and books written on the subject. A good multivitamin plus some extra vitamin A will suffice.

Add to this the very important action of breathing properly There are several ways to breathe. For normal passive everyday living, just fill your lungs every time you inhale completely. Before you tell me it is impossible to think about breathing every moment of the day, refer to the use of the method described in the chapter on the mind to develop a subliminal state of conscience. It will be of great assistance. At first, it is a lot of conscious repetitive action. Soon it will become second nature. Even when you do forget to do the necessary, your mind will remind you from time to time. The times when you become conscious of the necessity to breathe will balance with the time you do not think about breathing, and that will already register a big improvement compared to the way you used to breathe.

Another way is to breathe very deeply, at least once a day, ten times by forcing the shoulders back and pushing the stomach out, with the same movement using the diaphragm to suck the lungs full of air. Athletes should do that all the time. You will be surprised how much more energy will be yours for the taking. This was the most powerful tool in my box of tricks when climbing mountains, to get to the top and still be in a condition envied by some of my fellow climbers who used the more conventional methods of breathing. I must confess I very seldom let on what I was up to.

It is amazing how little nutrition the body needs to prosper in comparison to anything else that requires fuel to operate. The lungs are exceptional We do not need to add any fuel, they only require oxygen. We supply the oxygen and the lungs will deliver, all leading to an improved lifestyle that creates much more satisfaction only made possible when we push ourselves a little and make the effort. To enjoy the feeling of elation produced by endorphins coursing through the veins must be experienced to be appreciated.

Breath, breath, breath, deeeeeeply often.

OXYGEN IS LIFE. How long can a person live without oxygen? Not very long... a few minutes before brain damage sets in, then not many minutes more before the person stops breathing altogether. Some heart attacks can be stopped only by rapidly administering oxygen. Muscles cannot operate without oxygen. Does that not indicate the important role oxygen plays in keeping the body operating? If the lack of it can have such a dramatic effect on life itself, in such a short space of time, it seems to be the most important nutrient of all. Once again, I am bowled over by the indifference the human race displays towards the wonders of the amazing living body that we so blatantly taken for granted. Perhaps this will make them sit up and take note of the difference between what ***life is like and what it could be like***

I often walk up twenty-one floors while my breathing increases marginally. I ascribe it wholly to correct breathing and good nutrition as well as being reasonably fit. Nothing more earth-shattering.

Smoking is not probably, not arguably, but definitely the number one curse in the life of the smoker, and to a varied degree, the non-smoker. In my estimation, ninety-five percent of smokers would like to kick the diabolical habit, but cannot do it on account of a lack of willpower, discipline, and mind control. When you ask them why they don't stop smoking, the answer is always, "I can give it up whenever I choose to," but they still smoke. The alternative answer is, "I've tried every possible way to give up smoking, none of them works for me." Having asked this question and received this reply, some time later the same people develop complications with their health and when told by a physician to give up smoking or else, they do it instantly with no effort at all.

The dangers of smoking are well-documented so let's look at the put offs: the nauseating smell on their breath, and on their person. Smoking in one's car and one's home, often when they don't even smoke at that moment, still leaves the offensive smell lingering on for far longer than is desirable.

Smoking in one's private environment is a distinct invasion of one's privacy that does not seem to bother many smokers. They deem it their own divine right to do so. Such blatant lack of respect and disregard for the miracle of life, the care, and maintenance of this magnificent creation, the human body which they received free, gratis, and for nothing, is not possible to understand. For those who are genuinely serious about quitting the diabolical habit, there is hope, as described elsewhere. Mind control, weaning yourself from the dependence upon smoking cigarettes, and most important the attitude towards the miracle of life and gratitude towards your Creator.

Chapter 9

SINUS

The sinuses are found in the cavities above, between, and underneath the eyes next to the nose, and act as a safety net, together with the hairs in the nose, to trap and catch dust and impurities from entering among others, the lungs. It protects the mucous membrane, which is found all over the body and keeps it in good condition. These are just some of the many functions the sinus performs in the body that concerns us at this moment.

In the chapter on "Detoxing," the importance of keeping the body clean on the inside is discussed, and the same care is essential to ensure that the mucous membrane stays in a healthy condition to avoid infection. It is the lungs' first line of defense, consequently, the body's as well. So much can go wrong with your sinus on account of the enormous pollution problem we are forced to live with. There is no escaping the consequences. Performing a cleansing action like eating copious amounts of fruit and raw vegetables, as well as alternatively taking some herbal cleanser, will return a labouring sinus back to a healthy condition.

We can help a great deal by lending a hand and assist the sinus in the fight to keep the body healthy by becoming interested and paying closer attention to our health early in life, the earlier the better. To learn how to maintain a strong young healthy body from the word go is so much easier and more effective than learning the same later in life.

Another way to solve sinus problems is to run salt water through the sinus once or twice a year to prevent problems from developing. The best way to accomplish this is to use seawater. For those living inland where that is simply not an option, salt water solution made from ordinary table salt will suffice.

Mix a mild solution of table salt and water. Try a little first to make sure the solution is not too strong. Cup the hand, fill it with salt water, close one nostril with a finger and suck as much water into the sinus as high up into the nose as possible. Repeat the procedure with the other nostril. Go about your business as usual, only do not lean forward, or the salt water will run out of your nose and that is not what you want to happen. Keep the cavities full of water for as long as possible. It is busy doing what you want it to do, processing the mucous and getting it ready to be removed from where it has been sitting, perhaps for a very long time.

Salt has its uses around the house, for instance cleaning and sterilizing purposes like rinsing vegetables to be eaten raw, and for consumption as seldom as possible.

The body is designed to take care of the excess mucous in a natural way via the draining tubes, provided we do not interfere with nature as we humans are inclined to do, by consuming unnatural products in excess.

During the next day or two, the mucous that has been accumulating in the mucous membrane will start evacuating itself. Do not be surprised at the amount of mucous that will be expelled (depending how long since the mucous was last removed from the sinus). If never before, it can be substantial, sometimes resembling pieces of rubber.

To remove the excess mucous: in the distant past a ceramic device was used very successfully called the Sinus Pedi. It had a body resembling an oilcan, just much smaller, with a long spout, also smaller, and a small opening that fitted neatly into the nostril. One would fill the container with salt water, tilt the head to one side over a basin, put the spout into the upper nostril and pour very slowly, and surprise, surprise, the mixture comes out the other nostril. Repeat the process from the other side.

It may be possible to find one of these handy little gadgets somewhere. What a pity we have moved so far away from an holistic way of life. In the past these devices were available everywhere, now only good fortune will provide you with one.

One can perform such simple but very necessary tasks at home instead of having to visit the doctor, and more than likely have prescribed remedies, where a more natural way surely would have been a better choice.

Preferring natural holistic remedies should always be the first option, so much cheaper, no waiting for a doctor's appointment. With medical costs soaring, you may even get a bonus from your grateful medical insurance at the end of the year for not spending the society's money unnecessarily.

Athletes who practice any sport that involves seawater seldom have sinus problems.

An easy way to steer clear of one particular problem that affects the mucous membrane much more than one is inclined to think, is to avoid the mucous in cow's milk. It is so much more powerful and extremely harsh on the mucous membrane. The two are simply not compatible.

The sinus is part of the mucous membrane, and the mucous membrane needs nutrition. The food it likes the most is vitamin A, together with a combination of other vitamins and minerals.

To further do what we can to keep the mucous membrane in a healthy condition is to avoid drinking fresh cow's milk as far as possible. Boiling milk is one way to remove the heavy mucous, as well as processing the milk into products, for instance yogurt, cheese, or any other dairy product.

We are the only mammals that drink milk, even to a ripe old age after having been weaned. Milk is meant for calves and not for human consumption, a huge difference.

In the poorer areas where milk is usually easily available, little children often suffer heavy mucous discharge from the nose. For their families it is relatively easy to keep a cow or two and milk is regarded as good nutrition, which may be true, but the downside rules raw milk out as such. There is no sense in trying to keep children healthy, while at the same time creating other health problems.

The occasional head cold, which could probably also be avoided by practicing good nutrition, is a reasonably natural occurrence. The often or continuous experience of suffering head colds, or what may seem to be head colds, may very well be the sinus that has become infected by the use of raw cow milk and milk products. This possibility should be investigated. Attacks on the unhealthy sinus are a very painful experience and can sometimes be serious, remedy? Try nature first, go the salt treatment route. A case of lactose intolerance could also be the culprit. Curtailing the consumption of all dairy products for at least some time will quickly prove the theory correct or otherwise.

Calcium is a dire necessity in the diet, but calcium in excessive amounts, as is the case with milk, can also create problems.

Keep to a natural regime to maintain a natural balance. Enough calcium can be had from fresh leafy green vegetables and many other natural foods, for instance, cheese, molasses, and a diet of fresh fruit and vegetables. As an alternative, a multivitamin/mineral supplement that should include magnesium, another essential mineral combination with calcium, will take care of that little necessity.

A word of caution about molasses. Although a very healthy natural product with extremely high iron content, it is the remedy to take should one show signs of anemia. If the blood pressure is normal and no anemic condition exists, rather desist from taking molasses as it can increase the blood pressure. An excellent and absolutely safe remedy for an anemic condition called tissue salts is available from any health food store.

Molasses is another example of man's interference with nature to provide another by-product when refining sugar to create white sugar. Natural unrefined or partly refined sugar, like treacle for instance, is permissible to take in reasonable quantities.

Chapter 10

NERVES

The organ that controls not only the body in its entirety to the extent that, should it not be adequately cared for, disaster will overtake not only the body, but in a wider sense the person's whole and complete lifestyle.

The nerve system has two enemies: Stimulants, such as the abuse of caffeine, the most dangerous of all. It can cause unstable and out of control emotional conditions and situations.

Nervous breakdown! The first picture the mind conjures up when nerves are under discussion. (I call it by this name to make it easier for the layman to understand. The professionals prefer to call each of several conditions by its proper title. This book is for the lay person in layman's language, not only to make it easier to understand, but also so the reader does not become bored too quickly, which can happen easily when a person does not understand terms and names of what is under discussion). Initially, there does not appear to be damage of a physical nature, except that the person is severely distraught and emotionally stressed. That creates the impression that the problem is not at all physical.

The condition starts as an emotional problem and when it has developed far enough, the physical body becomes severely affected and the signs of severe stress the person is subjected to, becomes apparent. The nerve network covers the whole body, every muscle, organ, down to the root of every hair. Wherever one can feel the prick of a needle, there is a nerve ending present.

The nerve system is divided into several different sections, each with its own nerve center and name. *For instance, the sciatic nerve at the back of the leg, or the ulna nerve in the arm, among others.* Nerves are made up of very real tissue, although the cells of this particular kind are different to ordinary body cells. The nerves resemble telephone cables, from as thick as a grown man's small finger to the tiniest of threads that are not visible to the naked eye. When one of the larger nerves is cut through we find what resembles a large telephone cable filled with smaller cables. These cables or nerves consist of sensory nerves and motor nerves. The sensory nerves communicate touch sensation to the brain, while the brain instructs movement via the motor nerves to activate the muscles.

This is just another example of how extraordinary the body is. Imagine how fine the nerves at the tip of the finger are, and how sensitive touch is to that finger. So fine and yet they go to every cell in the skin over the entire body.

Any person who has had the experience of cutting through a nerve, for instance one in a finger, will know how unpleasant it can be to have lost feeling in the end of the finger where the tissue is completely dead. Nerves do grow, and most of the time the cut nerve endings find each other. The sensory nerve finds the sensory nerve and the same for the motor nerve. It does take a very long time to grow together, as the nerve cells being different to other cells grow extremely slowly. For some time the feeling in that part of the finger will be gone, leaving a rather unpleasant sensation. For instance, picking up something off the floor can be a strange experience, or touching any other part of the body with that finger takes getting used to.

The nerves resemble telephone cables and when they are in operation are just as direct and instant. Touch something and it registers instantly in the brain, not only the touch but also the particular texture of the object you touched, which makes it possible to distinguish one object from literally a million others, even the difference in thickness of one and two sheets of paper.

The nerves can become diseased just like any other part of the body. Consider for a moment the incredible stress and tension the average person is subjected to during just one day. The stress is, of course, not registered in the nervous system but in the brain. The brain is then obliged to react according to what it was instructed to do, and it does that via the nervous system. Imagine a severely stressful situation. The whole body is involved, the glands, every single muscle, organ, tendon; they are all connected into one vast network, the nerve system.

The whole body and all it contains are under stress, and the nerves suffer an overload on account of being the communication network. One can understand what happens with the nerve system when you compare it to a similar system outside the body. An electrical or telephone network that is overloaded when the demand outstrips the capacity, self-destructs, or in modern terms a safety switch is activated. The nervous system does not have a safety fuse. Our safety mechanism is self-control, and if for some reason or the other we do not practice self-control, or on account of the enormous amount of stress modern day life demands, it cannot cope, and it simply overheats.

The capacity and resilience of the nerves to handle stress is remarkable, unfortunately not without limitations. When tension reaches boiling point the whole person suffers and we have a total breakdown on our hands. Virtually every component in the body is affected. The glands that excrete different chemicals throughout the entire body are out of control, and the stomach with all its different acids and chemicals experience a severe state of disorder. It is tantamount to a chemical war that has erupted inside the body. Soon the whole system will be in chaos, with the nerves being the worst affected.

When this sad scenario gets out of control to the extent described above and the nerves "snap" for want of a better word, it is usually a disaster of major proportions and will take a long time and much effort to get the system back on track and a semblance of normality. For the nerves, and consequently the whole person, to be the same as before the catastrophe struck can take years of hard work and dedication. Unfortunately, often depending on the severity of the case, a complete cure is not possible. The person will have a severe "hangover" that can leave him/her vulnerable to any situation that is not completely stable for the rest of their life, which will make a completely normal life almost impossible.

As stated previously the nerve system has several different "nerve centers," the main one being situated in the center of the stomach, and the conditions described above in the stomach affects the nerve center situated there most severely, so severely that it is almost impossible to eat. The nerves are extremely sensitive and vulnerable at this stage and are present everywhere throughout the stomach and control, among other things, the muscles in the stomach. They are not capable of performing their functions in a normal fashion, or in severe cases not at all. When one does not eat, one becomes weak. Add to that the fact that it is almost impossible to sleep due to the fact that it is in the brain where chaos now reigns, where the problem first manifested. For that person life is on hold in a very unpleasant way.

All muscle tissues are affected, and the deterioration in the condition of the body as a whole is traumatic. Nothing escapes these traumatic conditions and an upset of this magnitude causes the normal operation of life more often than not, to come to a standstill. If you can picture a person experiencing such a catastrophe in his/her life, then you can understand why a nerve "breakdown" is such a serious event, with consequences that most of the time result in major interruptions of ordinary life, often for a very long time.

Healing must take place first of all in the mind where it started, and that is usually a long and slow process. I have been told by an expert that in the case of a severe breakdown the chances of regaining *complete* recovery and control of the nervous system is very small, and should that happen the individual will be extremely fortunate. It will in most cases leave the individual with fragile nerves that will need tender loving care on a permanent basis.

A condition of this nature should, if possible, be avoided at all cost. This may sound a bit dramatic, and it certainly is no exaggeration. This is meant to be a warning because it can be extremely serious. When conditions become severe, and it is simply not possible to slow down the pace or move away from a stressful situation, the best advice would be to increase the intake of vitamin B to maximum quantities. This will have a cushioning effect, but will not solve the problem. A person as a whole is simply not designed to operate under such extreme conditions.

Healing is slow and arduous. It is possible for life to continue in a normal way, usually only after a long period of counseling and the inevitable administering of drugs. Do not worry and do not rebel. Take the drugs. There is light at the end of the tunnel and the best thing is, simply to do as suggested by the professional under whose care you will find yourself by now.

It is almost certain that the drugs prescribed will be habit-forming. Don't stress, when the time comes that you feel you can begin to relinquish the support and comfort these drugs offer, simply wean yourself off them by dividing one of the tablets into four quarters and take one-quarter less every four or five days. It is time-consuming but worth the wait, and with discipline is absolutely fool-proof.

This is where holistic healing becomes your ally. If you have not been introduced to them before, vitamins become your friends. Yes, the trusted vitamin B steps to the fore. Take a multivitamin that contains large doses of vitamin B, which will become your mainstay. There are several B vitamins. Don't be concerned, they will be correctly formulated. If you are already taking a multivitamin, add an additional high dose of vitamin B to the mix.

Your nerves may be suspect for a long time to come, or perhaps the damage was so severe that you may have to take these vitamins for the rest of your life. Although your nerves will more than likely still be vulnerable, you will at least to all intents and purposes feel completely normal. Should you wish to stop taking the vitamins, do it at a slow pace as you could suffer vitamin deficiency syndrome. You will soon know whether it was the right thing to do. It is advisable to take a multivitamin on a regular basis in any event. Vitamin B is an expensive remedy, but unfortunately, you have no alternative other than drugs, which are not advisable. They are not natural and can cause serious problems in the long run, including the danger of permanent addiction. Vitamins will have many other healthy and beneficial spin-offs, which in this case may be paid for by medical insurance.

There is another negative spin-off that can occur should one be reckless and disregard the warnings of a previously traumatized nerve system, and that is called shingles. Shingles are extremely painful and are all physical, ***involving one entire nerve section.*** The particular section becomes infected, and usually involves a complete section of the nerve system in the body, for instance, the sciatic nerve that runs over the buttocks and down the rear of the leg.

Another goes over the side of the head and the face, this particular one can be so severe that it can affect the eyesight and cause permanent eye damage. Either condition is painful and uncomfortable and can last for what seems like an eternity. The external appearance can be horrific as the whole nerve section, right to the smallest ends, are infected. It forms a thick scab over the whole area, which can cover the size of a dinner plate. This condition is not permanent and one usually recovers completely. The treatment is extremely expensive. *It is all avoidable, but be on guard at all times and don't think it can't happen to you. The effects are insidious and you could be in for a rude awakening.*

One way to bolster the defenses and minimize the effects of such a tragic event is to maintain a holistic lifestyle. That will bolster the capacity of the whole body to fight off attacks of all kinds.

The major common enemy of nerves is the destructive effect caffeine has on the nerve system. It is common for heavy coffee drinkers to be tense, pent up, stressed out, etc. Their lives are in turmoil, and they blame their nervous condition on the problems they are experiencing, which can eventually lead to a nerves breakdown. In actual fact, the sad state of their affairs is due to the poor condition their nerves are in, which in turn are due to the heavy caffeine intake. It all started with drinking too much coffee. (AMONG OTHERS) There is an answer to the problem – caffeine-free coffee, it tastes just as good.

MORAL OF THE STORY: TRY AND PRE EMPT AND AVOID A BREAKDOWN AT ALL COST.

BOOK TWO

Chapter 11

MIND DYNAMICS

"AS MAN THINKETH SO IS HE"

Achieve eternal success by the way you think. Your whole life, past, present and future, will be registered in your mind. Learn how to control your mind. Turn it on or off at will and you will be in control of your life. What power, what freedom!

Is good nutrition essential for the optimum functioning of the brain? I would say without a doubt, yes, like the body it is made up of tissue, albeit different. As in the body, the cells die and break down and need to be repaired and replaced, a job only nutrition can do.

The brain – this is where all activities are directed from that concern and influences life. That makes it an awesome instrument, the only one of its kind. What makes the brain, and you, so powerful are the power you have over the mind. This is the area in a physical brain, among several other divisions, that is not physical and where thinking takes place. Thoughts are not physical, they are ethereal and this is where they are transformed to become physical. Is that not awesome? So incredible, no limitations as to what can be achieved. The sky is the limit (guess where the ideas of great inventions were conceived).

Whatever your mind can conceive and believe, you will be able to achieve.

Before we can enjoy all these wonderful riches the mind, body, and soul can deliver, we have to learn and understand how it all works to deliver these amazing and positive results. The mind, the body, and the soul – a very common expression, but there is more to it than merely these three. There is the individual as well, the person.

All of them are encapsulated in the brain plus the memory, conscience, and sub-conscience. They all play a vital role in the execution of every single thought and action that comes to fruition as we will see later on.

The sum total that makes life a reality, the force that is responsible for the tremendous successes that are achieved, that is generally accepted, but who does the planning? Not the mind, as is so commonly accepted, there is another force at play here – the person who is in control and he/she instructs the mind accordingly.

At the same time, at the other end of the scale the mind can be left to do without direction as we commonly believe, and is so often the case. What it automatically does without direction or interference from a control centre, runs the affairs of and controls the brain, which in turn controls the body with, at best, mediocre results.

To understand how the "person" influences life and makes possible the sweet taste of success, which is not reserved for the privileged few only but for everybody, needs to be explained. Understanding how this all works together involves the person, mind, body, and soul, that create the personality that each of us presents to the world. It must begin somewhere, and that is not with the brain nor the mind, but an understanding of the theory that the person is in control. Understanding this theory makes understanding the principle of positive thinking so much easier, which is so essential to creating a positive mindset, the only path to success.

For anybody who wants to enjoy success, and perhaps through no fault of his or her own has not had the opportunity or the understanding to make it happen, and perhaps been made to believe that it is simply not possible for them to achieve success, there is some good news. If he or she is a member of the "average person" category, he/she only needs to be taught to understand the statement above in order to enjoy their share of success and ultimate joy and happiness. It is possible, for anybody of average intelligence also to be "fortunate" by learning **what is and how a positive mind can and must be developed. Read on.**

There is a way to change that negative frame of mind, to blow the artificially imposed ceiling sky high, to remove the fences, the barriers, anything that will prevent that person from emulating the success of others. It is possible to break through the invisible walls that surround their minds, and that is easier than what is generally accepted. By learning to think outside the box, and with the correct guidance, tuition and motivation, together with just one small success, the tiny little snowball will start to move. That education to self-empowerment starts with the person himself.

Here the person will be taken at his own pace to learn and understand what the statement above entails, and realize that it is possible to enjoy a better lifestyle and that it is really not difficult. No formal education is required. It starts with gaining enough confidence to believe in oneself, and the confidence usually comes with understanding. No matter at what stage that person's level of confidence is, once he/she has been exposed to the theories herein and with enough willpower and determination, a certain amount of belief will have been achieved to make the beginning of success possible. If a person can read, he or she can become educated in this very natural or any other skill.

Let's delve a little deeper and seek some understanding of the whole process.

Who is in control of our lives? We are, the person, you yourself, l myself, not the mind. The mind has no control or jurisdiction over the person.

We decide and instruct the mind what it will think; **we** decide what we want out of life, and only then do we employ our mind to do the thinking that is required to bring about the fulfillment of our wishes. To be able to do that, we need to learn how that is made possible.

To make it easy to understand the workings of the whole process, let us separate the whole into four different entities – the person, mind, soul, and the body. The last three are of course encapsulated in the brain, which has many different divisions.

Become acquainted with the awesome power of the mind, a disciplined mind, a power you are in control of and is directed by you (more of this in the chapter on discipline.) This is where it all happens, where it is decided whether your future will turn out to be a success, a failure, or somewhere in between. Any one of those can be your future companion. Any average person can achieve exactly what he or she believes they can achieve. Unfortunately, if no conscience choice is made, one of the last two futures mentioned is what will happen to most people. Conditions or circumstances decide for them, often inadvertently. What motivates people to make a choice or not to make a choice... a lack of discipline, shear laziness, perhaps ignorance, a negative background, a lack of motivation, or simply fear of the unknown?

No matter what the reason, success is possible for the vast majority and it is easier than one may think. Success is not restricted to only a few fortunate individuals. It is for anybody who is of average intelligence, which comprises ninety percent of the population. Those who were fortunate enough to become disciplined and learned to think constructively, have found the necessary source of information, and are willing to make the effort to empower himself or herself, can achieve financial success, a successful social life, and will inevitably become happy and contented as a reward. Not all successful people are necessarily "more intelligent." They were if anything, a lot more fortunate at learning or at discovering the secret. Often it is no secret that the person may be gifted with a retentive memory.

That does not make him/her more intelligent. They still have to learn how to think and that being academically gifted does not mean automatic success, a very common misconception and reason for failure. It is imperative that they acquire the very necessary skill – intellectual ability and that is achieved through constant <u>constructive</u> positive thinking

How does it work *in* practice? How does one go about understanding and learning what it is all about? After all, it is always easy when you know how things work or fit together.

Let's dig a little deeper and see if we can figure the workings of the mind.

"Take control of your life, or pull yourself together." Has anyone ever thought what those words which are so liberally bandied about actually mean in graphic detail? Who must take control of what, or what must take control of what? According to the way I understand along conventional lines of thinking, this is not possible. In those terms, the "you" referred to consists of mind, body, and soul, so there is nothing to pull or take. After all, it does not work together as a single unit. Now, let's look at the whole creative process from this more simplified or easier to understand angle.

Separate the person, who is after all in charge of the creative process of the mind, which is where the conscious and subconscious are found. Each one of these has a separate function to perform. In the case of a disciplined person, he decides what the mind should think and how it should think and remember, not only positive, it could be negative as well. He, the person becomes the decision maker. One can almost say, a "dictator" to the mind. The mind being subservient to the person, without argument accepts what has been decided upon. The mind is instructed what the thinking should entail. That is when dialogue is initiated between the mind and the person. This takes place instantaneously. Nothing works faster than the brain.

It is important for the "person" to understand and realize there is a separation **and that he is in charge** of the mind. To become effective, this must happen on a regular basis by making a concerted effort to remember to take charge, until it becomes a habit and eventually a characteristic of one's personality. That is how a powerful and disciplined mind is created. It will not happen overnight. Time, patience, and practice are required for the mind to accept the change and learn to operate accordingly.

The mind can only work with material obtained from the subconscious. The subconscious is merely a store room of the accumulated material. Hence the importance of the quality of the material the person allows the subconscious to accumulate via the five senses, positive or negative, creative or otherwise. It becomes clear how important the role the person plays in determining the quality of his life by controlling the quality of material, positive or negative, the subconscious accepts and absorbs at random which the mind then feeds off. That is how we become disciplined thinkers. There is a lot more to what we know about the process known as "to think." ***Thus it is clear that the more knowledge the subconscious accumulates, the more beneficial it will be to achieve success.***

Once again, for reasons of easy understanding, imagine that the thinking process is a dialogue between the person and the mind. After all, that is what we do all day long. When we think, we literally talk to ourselves, silently of course. At least now that we understand a little more, it does not seem so embarrassing. We and our minds interact through dialogue continuously. The only difference is that we have now learned to think positively and constructively. We have the choice to daydream or not. That choice belongs to us. It is now much easier to understand the process, and how to adopt a positive attitude and become a positive person, by the person controlling the mind and not allowing the mind to fall into negative mode.

In a life that has been operating without the person directing the course of events, the mind is usually undisciplined and life, in general, is a very unhappy one.

Where life is completely out of control, one can say there is no direction and the whole process works from the bottom up. In other words, the senses are in charge. Whatever appeal to the senses is accepted or simply happens, there is no direction or discipline, with consequential results.

Apart from hard work, not much in the line of academic qualifications are needed to give the underprivileged person a chance to have a shot at success, other than to learn how to develop, use, and operate a disciplined mind.

The secret is to motivate and make the average person aware of the possibility of enjoying a better life, and realizing there is hope for them as well. How is that achieved? Learn to think in a disciplined and orderly manner and empower yourself to achieve eventual success.

Learn to become a thinker and become addicted to the awesome power of thought and your mind will automatically be in thinking mode without much effort or prompting from your side. A successful end result will be so powerful it will liberate your thinking process and give you enormous freedom.

The more you practice what you learn, the more your mind will be in top gear and stay there. Your mind is disciplined to observe any action, opportunity, or object, out of the ordinary that holds promise to be turned into a successful venture that would pass by other less disciplined minds. Think for a moment what that entails, what an advantage you hold. Your senses become far sharper than the average non-thinking, or perhaps even thinking person. Yes! You have moved up a rung or two on the ladder towards success. Your brain begins to work differently. An overheard conversation, something you may have read in some magazine or newspaper, triggers a new and different line of thought, and the opportunities and possibilities to grow are endless. When you learn to think rationally, you and your mind learn to communicate as the common expression indicates, "two minds are better than one." Imagine how powerful that can b. It is what we do all day long – dialogue – every moment we are awake, just in a more controlled manner with better understanding. No more day-dreaming. That has now become "controlled thinking." We are exercising the mind continuously, hence it becomes stronger all the time.

Dislodge yourself from what is considered by many to be normal conditions, situations, or surroundings, in other words, a boring existence found in a stultified environment. Learn to see the wood from the trees, recognize the possibilities and make them work for you, smarter not harder.

We hold our destiny in our own hand. We have the right to decide for ourselves what we want out of life, and no other person has the right to try and dominate us or influence our thoughts against our will. Empower yourself, discover your true potential.

The most successful thief of self-respect, success, prosperity, and anything that is positive, are negative preconceived ideas that we have about ourselves. The reason? Most of the time the way we have been raised to think, which is not necessarily a bad thing *per se*, is that our parents have merely attempted to make us decent and respectable citizens. *What they failed to do, unfortunately, is to administer the antidote – explain the difference between being just "ordinary" and being positive and developing our potential to be the best we can be and still be solid citizens.* If that is the case with you, then it is vitally important that you follow these instructions carefully and develop your mind to its full potential without feeling guilty.

I believe success is inevitable, provided you are determined to win in the end. It goes without saying that one has to be realistic, and not allow day-dreaming to influence our thinking. It is a fact that whatever your mind, as directed by you, can conceive and **believe,** it will be able to achieve. I believe I can go in any direction and with dedication and a positive mindset, and conquer any project successfully that I **believe** can be brought to a successful conclusion.

We all have more or less the same capacity brainpower. It is the limitations we place upon ourselves, mostly unwittingly, that blocks success. Remove those limitations. Success is not reserved for the fortunate few and even if that were the case, then believe that you are one of the few. Go out there and get whatever your heart desires, it is rightfully yours.

To believe that you are mediocre or just "ordinary" is to do you a gross injustice. Nothing ordinary has ever excelled and that translates into no success in any direction. That is not what you desire for yourself.

Listen to advice. Be careful, you be the judge and decide for yourself if any intended influence is to your advantage and of positive value. You decide. Do not be intimidated, or afraid to walk away from any decision made on your behalf that you do not agree with once you have empowered yourself and have the courage to disagree with anybody, should you wish to. From now on, you are the master of your own fate, designer of the kind of soul you wish to have for yourself, with a lifestyle to match, a respected member of any community to which you wish to make a positive contribution. After all, it is the soul that matters. That is where genuine satisfaction, contentment, and happiness, ultimately manifest themselves and are expressed through us and become our personality, which is the essence of life.

The positive effect will be felt on a much wider scale than merely by you. It will touch other people's lives in a positive way as well. That does not mean that advice should be discarded without it being looked at carefully, especially that of older people who have walked the road and know the pitfalls. *A wise old mind together with a vibrant young one makes for a powerful combination.*

Now comes the fun part. Prepare to meet what will turn out to be the most enjoyable and pleasant experience of your life.

Your mind becomes your closest friend, best buddy, and confidant. Think about the fact that you and your mind dialogue continuously all day long (internal dialog) and exchange thoughts every moment you are awake. Your mind never stops thinking, and that is where the hidden power lies, in organized thought. Once you have become disciplined, you have the power to change the direction your mind is traveling should you disagree. This is the power that gives birth to new ideas you the person will nurture, make to grow and expand, and lead to unbridled happiness.

At night it is a little different. Your conscious mind is asleep, while your subconscious mind is still active. That is when you dream. Sometimes we talk out loud during a careless moment, nothing wrong with that, although it may create the wrong impression with people who do not understand how the mind works, or where in life you happened to be at that moment. You have moved on. They may not have, a big difference should they still operate in the old-fashioned way. Take no notice, you are in charge. That is an indication that you, the person, is in total control of the whole process that is taking place in the brain, very productive and most of all positive. Don't let what people think disturb you, as long as you know what your thinking is all about and that you are in control.

Sometimes it is necessary to be, or appear to be a loner. Don't allow it to bother you.

Loneliness will not easily be a bugbear in your life from now on. One's thoughts can be wonderful companions, provided they are positive and constructive. Have no fear of becoming a solitary soul that prefers only your own company, far from it. You will become so curious about all that is happening around you, life will take on a completely different meaning. You will want to hear all that other people say and put your own individual slant on matters. You are becoming an individual thinker and listener. Out come? Loneliness is no longer a threat.

At this stage it is best not to divulge too much about your newly found powers. Rather relish the success in the privacy of your personal being. The time will come when you will be more in control of what you have learned and then make worthwhile contributions.

Something interesting may happen to you at this stage. You may become very interested in the conversations you hear going on around you. You may tend to just listen and evaluate what is said without making comment. This is another way of broadening your outlook and learning by putting your own slant on what you hear. This will exercise your thinking ability. Take care not to become anti-social, a smart ass, always knowing better. Always maintain your dignity. You have one mouth and two ears. Use them in the same ratio. It is called discipline.

The mind will become addicted to any thought you the person will allow. *Negative thoughts usually happen insidiously. You are not even aware of what is occurring, unless you have progressed far enough in the thought controlling process to become aware of it taking place and you can put a stop to it immediately. Why not become addicted to thinking positive, constructive thoughts? Not only is it an enormous amount of fun, it puts you in a very powerful position. Nothing in life stays constant or is static. If it does not progress, it regresses. Thinking is no different. Think positive all the time, which should be by now an automatic process, and you will remain positive.*

It is a growing process from small beginnings, little by little, until your mind becomes a tiny mental juggernaut. You will be building continuously and are creating a very powerful entity – you. Ever thought it could happen to you? Believe me, it can. Your mind is a mind like any other. Equally, so the thought process is like any other process of any kind, you can develop and make it grow.

Only positive thoughts will create positive thoughts. Negative thoughts are by definition negative and have no constructive contribution to make. See how important it is to stay away from the negative in all aspects of life? The same power is behind them and has an equal opportunity to destroy. Don't be drawn into arguments, be your own person, walk away from anything negative. You cannot afford to be distracted at this stage while you are growing, be careful with whom you discuss what you are learning. The area of practice will become so wide it will influence your whole existence and you will eventually practice the wisdom and knowledge you will have gained wherever, whenever and however you choose to. Inevitably, you will become curious about many subjects and you will want to know more about them. This will lead to developing the educational side, for instance, reading, researching the internet etc. Gaining and accumulating knowledge will become addictive and happen automatically. Knowledge is power. Nothing holds more power than a well-thought outspoken word.

Consider the following. Imagine you are locked up in solitary confinement for many years, (pray it will never happen) as has happened often before to many people. The average person without this kind of training will be fortunate to remain sane or even survive. With your ability to control your thinking, engaged in positive mode you would not only survive, but could actually prosper. You will be able to separate yourself from any condition or circumstance within the confines you find yourself in. By conceiving ideas and with disciplined thinking, actually expand and build upon those ideas, you can complete huge projects without even as much as writing down one single sentence, all in the confines of your own mind. Not only will your mind be exercised and grow during this process, your memory will do likewise, growing beyond all expectations.

There is no computer in existence that is as powerful as the mind, for one simple reason, we can think and there is no limit to the amount of knowledge that the memory can store. You can tackle as many projects as you wish, they will always be available for you to retrieve from your memory. It may take a little prompting sometimes, no problem, one thought will lead to another. Allow your mind to dwell on the subject in question and it will soon fall into place. Just think how much fun you will have once you have mastered the art of controlling your thinking and your memory.

There are several kinds of thinking. One is when you explore thoughts while alone; another is during conversations, when you study, technical thinking is when you decipher a complexity of sorts. No matter what your thoughts are, they will exercise your mind provided they are positive and constructive.

Challenges. In the world of mediocrity this word usually conjures up something that is best left to someone else. It sounds like hard work, and can sometimes be scary. To the motivated person, the one you should be by now or soon will be, the word will create a feeling of excitement with a capital 'E'. Should you still see goals as huge mountains of frightening proportions staring you in the face, not to worry this will soon change. It is amazing how quickly things can turn around from the negative to the positive and you will be a winner. Then you will welcome any mountain of any size.

Some time or the other you will come across a problem that defies logic. Don't fuss, think about it thoroughly, file it away in your memory bank. It will receive attention you are not even aware of, and soon the answer will be at your fingertips. Your mind has been trained to handle eventualities without you being aware of it taking place.

There is nothing that makes the adrenaline flow faster than solving a problem or achieving success. No matter how small, it is exciting. Now move on to bigger challenges and before long, with the kind of insight you have gained, you will be a success or an adrenalin junkie, more than likely both. You will be looking for challenges. How will that be for motivation? Before long it will become a pleasant pastime and you will be looking for challenges to demolish. That is the way it was with me. I am still to meet the person that has a life as exciting as mine (not denying there are many; lives move on many levels and in many different directions). Believe it or not, I was once in the same category as the one you found yourself in before reading this, albeit a long time ago. There is nothing I enjoy as much as conceiving ideas about projects, planning, and executing those plans in my mind without as much as writing one line or word. I challenge myself to complete the whole project, from start to finish in this way. Sometimes even I am astonished at the size of the projects and the measure of success I achieve.

Assuming you have finished reading this chapter and have actually taken on the challenge to expand your mind, and it is some time since you started this journey, is it becoming clear how much your mind has developed and expanded with only the application of positive thoughts and effort? Compare that to what your mind was like only a short while ago. As I said before, it is possible for any person who feels uncertain within himself, to eventually be successful. Start by taking one thought at a time. You **will soon achieve** whatever your mind can conceive **and** believe. You give direction and the mind will follow. In the life of the unsuccessful person, the mind is in control and not the person, and it is a case of the blind leading the blind.

There are other areas where a positive attitude can bring about a huge difference in a person's life; emotionally for instance, or eradicating some bad habits gained during a period of insecurity or lack of confidence, or "following the pack" syndrome. The person has now, with a new positive outlook on life, realized there is a better way to find confidence by becoming an independent thinker, which will open up a new world for him that he could never have imagined possible. No more relying on wisdom from others to set the pace. Life consists of many different facets. Take a look and see what you have learned up till now, it will work in practice where other aspects of life are also involved. Let's look at some of these aspects.

Life is full of unwanted habits. Should you be a victim and you would like to make a change, now you can. You have more confidence and the capacity to make change. Nothing is stopping you from taking the first step to becoming a gigantic success. Accept it as a challenge.

You have to start somewhere, so try something easy. Now you have learned how to empower yourself, start putting it into practice. Begin by changing some worrying aspect of your life brought about by negative thinking. Select one that you think is the least of your worries, but which you would like to change anyway. How does one eat an elephant? One small bite at a time! The secret is repetition, rather than trying to change the situation as quickly as possible. It is a process of education, educating the mind in a new direction, a new process the mind is not used to. Remember, you are in charge; you make the decisions; the mind has learned to gladly follow suit and soon both of you will be empowered in a completely new way.

Let's begin with a nagging habit you would like to kick. Now is the time to start. Now that you have grasped the principle of mind control, you are excited at the prospect of using your new found power. In the beginning, it will need a lot of effort to constantly remind your mind to stop thinking in the negative. That will soon change. You will slowly become aware of the fact that negative thoughts are trying to prowl your thought process. Be ruthless and eradicate them immediately. Slowly your mind will accept the new way of thinking positively. The negative thoughts are overpowered and positive thinking has taken the commanding position in your mind and it will be the end of those bad habits. Your mind is so much more powerful and the old habit will become easier to handle and be banished from your mind.

By now it will not be difficult for you to dictate to your mind what the terms of reference are. All it takes is a little time and practice for your mind to accept the new rules that will give direction and meaning to your life. You are a new person. It takes time and effort, in other words, dedication and training. Look forward to the time when you are on par or have even overtaken those who in the past were seen by you as your superiors. Yes, we all have brain power in more or less equal measure. It is only a matter of effort and application that will put you in an advantaged position. Nothing can beat the sweet smell of success as a motivating factor.

Are there areas or instances where this system does not work where other personalities are involved? Yes, very few. One instance that comes to mind is according to Dr. Victor Frankl, the greatest psychologist of the twentieth century, who believed that there are some changes to emotional feelings in life that one cannot "will," for instance, love. You cannot will yourself to love someone or something. You can learn to accept that person. In a subtle way the mind needs to be trained or persuaded to accept the situation. After all, this is what civilization is based upon.

Once again, repetition is the answer. That goes for all universal thinking wherever it matters and not only love, which was merely an example. You cannot change the world on your own, but you can influence an opinion once your mind is well trained and the two of you understand each other well enough for you to become the dominant force in this powerful partnership you have created. After all, it is impossible for any organization or partnership to work where there are two entities in charge. One of them has to assume authority.

Lonely? You never again need to be lonely. You have a companion that is closer to you than hands and feet and, believe me, it is difficult to think of a more pleasant pastime than using your newly developed faculties. You will be too busy using them to realize that you are physically alone. Your mind will become a fertile source of new information. On account of the new way of thinking, your mind will automatically seek out new developments it can take on. Make it grow, expand and bring to fruition. It will become second nature to evaluate every new thought and observe what is happening around you.

The art of creation becomes so much easier to learn and adopt as part of your life and it is all based on positive thinking. ***Positive thoughts create more positive thoughts.*** You will find that new subjects come to mind all the time. Because of your new way of thinking, old ones you have discarded long ago are now looked at in a different light, hold new promise and are automatically reconsidered and rehashed. Schemes or projects that took on an air of impossibility in the past may now be seen through differently tinted glasses. That is so handy for entrepreneurs.

It will reach the stage where your mind will be tuned to investigating any situation that may hold promise to be exploited. Anything new the eye sees that may have a possibility of success will compel you to investigate further. Eventually, you may become so curious, you want to know how everything works, how they stick together, what makes them tick. This will inevitably lead you to develop an insatiable appetite for knowledge. A compulsion to investigate every opportunity, and automatically learn all there is to learn about any new idea, and so accumulate a vast amount of knowledge.

Developing an insatiable appetite for knowledge is one of the most satisfying experiences one can enjoy, and inevitably will become a potent source of new ideas in your life. Knowledge is power. The wider your knowledge, the wider the scope to come up with new ideas. In fact, the ideas will find you rather than you having to look for them. Ideas are always on the prowl looking for fertile minds. I can go on and on; where the mind is concerned, the sky is the limit.

It is clear that every person who falls within the brackets of average intelligence has an opportunity to succeed in life. All that is required is to understand and apply what is explained above. This is when it becomes clear that the average mind uses only a fraction of the power it possesses.

For example, consider an average mind that has been subjected to this kind of treatment. Minds grow the same way as muscles in the body. Put it under stress, in other words, use it, and it will become bigger and stronger by thinking positively on a regular basis, little by little. It does not have to be huge efforts, that will come later. Every positive thought will cause your faculties to grow. In other words, your mind, your memory, your whole mental ability, will expand.

There is no computer in existence that can be compared to the human brain. Is that not exciting? And that also includes *your* brain. You can do anything you put your new super brain too compared to what it was before. Believe in yourself. Liberated positive attitudes attract opportunities. Now that you think and see things differently, don't be surprised when you see possibilities, where in the past there was only opposition to anything that crossed your mind, thinking you could not do it or it was far above your ability. Destroy, delete, eradicate, and do anything you have to, to eliminate the words *"I CAN'T"* from your vocabulary. It no longer exists.

You are capable of being successful at anything your mind can conceive. ***Believe you can achieve it, and you will be able to***. The more positive you are, the easier the tasks that confront you will become. The solutions will be so much easier to spot and be understood. Remember, you have liberated your mind from the restrictions of the past, and you believe in yourself. That gives you so much power; your brain is now free to do what it has been designed to do – think, deliberate, plan, and so much more. No more restrictions – as long as you ***believe in yourself*** and maintain a positive attitude. Believe that you are on par with the rest and the best.

Develop a "go get it" attitude. If anyone else can get it or do it, so can you. It will not be long and you will beat them to it and the prize will be yours simply by thinking about it first, seeing it first, or recognizing possibilities others have missed. Because your newly acquired talents, you have become proactive instead of waiting in the background for something that was never going to happen, and now it is within touching distance. Remember, it is not the dog in the fight, but the fight in the dog that counts.

Your brain power is, with slight variations, the same as the next person. The only difference is **you are now in control.** No matter who you are, where you come from, what kind of background has shaped your life, what you look like, tall, thin, short or fat, it is the brain power that counts and there **we**, the average persons, all fall within the same category. Any person at any time uses only a fraction of their brain power. It does not take a genius to crack every nut in existence, anybody can do it provided they have made the effort to better prepare themselves. It all matters how **you** condition yourself. Nobody can do it for you. Go out there and just do it, no task is too big. As long as you believe you can conquer it, you will. I just love the slogan of a well-known and loved sports goods manufacturer, "just, do it." Guess why they are my favourite people.

New developments will take place in your life as your mind expands. Your life will be decidedly different and a whole lot more interesting. You may become more psychologically aware. *Where do we find the most interesting subjects in life? With human beings, of course! You may find you are more aware of what people say and do. The interest lies more in why they say and do things (psychology provides an enormous amount of fun.)*

Society does not approve of one person analyzing another. There is nothing wrong with analisyzing what they say and do though, it is a very interesting pastime. This should only take place in the privacy of your own mind. It has become an enormously interesting, shall I say a "hobby" it provides me with many hours of interesting discourses with myself and sometimes others (discretion recommended). You can learn so much about yourself while studying other people's behaviour and it does not stop there. My interest in history grew in leaps and bounds while reading about past leaders, how their thinking helped to shape the world we have inherited from them, and how our lives became what they are today, and inevitably I wonder how different could life have been, for better or worse.

The wider your knowledge on psychology, the easier it becomes to assess the attitude of people you have to deal with while deciding on business deals. We do not all get along with each other all the time from day to day. It can be crucial when you have to make the choice of a business partner, for example. That can be a make or break situation if you choose a partner whose personality clashes with your own. It would be wise to leave that little caper until you are well qualified to make the decision. Even if it looks like a once-in-a-lifetime opportunity (they do have the habit of making repeat appearances), it can leave you with scars that can take a very long time to heal and set you back financially and otherwise for some time to come.

There is an expression in the business world: a partnership is like marriage, the only difference; there is no sex. It is as important as choosing a marriage partner. You will be spending a lot of time together and some important decisions will have to be made. If you seldom agree on anything, it can be a long and cold winter.

It can be restrictive when you are in business alone to find time off for yourself or to attend to family matters, or whatever. Rather than look at partnerships, employ people you can trust. It will be cheaper in the long run. For a small business, there is always someone looking for part-time work that can do duty for you on an hourly basis.

Psychology is a huge subject and once it has aroused your curiosity and you have been bitten by the bug, it will take a mammoth effort to shake the habit. I am not so sure I want to do that, I find it not only enormously interesting to analyze people and their behavior, but also hugely beneficial, and adds to my repertoire of knowledge on different subjects, including myself.

A note of caution. Be careful not to start thinking at night, it may rob you of some sleep. It is so exciting once you start thinking, you do not want to stop. In the chapter on Insomnia you will learn how to handle that little problem of sleep, or rather, soothing the mind and making yourself fall asleep with consummate ease.

Serious and more difficult situations need the same treatment, but the desired change may take a little longer. For instance, smoking, a weight problem, over-indulgence etc. That will be as long as it takes to reprogram the mind, usually plus minus twenty-one days. Further on there are some more aids that can be employed, for instance, weaning, to help with the really difficult situations like smoking. Changing a habit by means of the thought process should by now be for you the most powerful and easiest way to change that bad habit.

In the all-powerful mind is where it all begins, and this is where fundamental change must take place to be permanent. Once the thinking process has been altered, the whole outlook changes. You, the all-powerful ally, constantly inform the mind what direction it should follow. It will soon start getting the message and slowly begin to change direction and turn its back on the old habit that has now lost out to the new way of thinking.

Your strong positive mind is now in control. You are now firmly in charge. When your mind tries to wander or transgress, bring it back into line. Be very firm, even ruthless. For instance, **make it clear that any tempting, irresistible thoughts are off limits, end of story, and that is final, forget it.** The trick is to treat your mind as a separate entity. Become a dictator, (to your mind only), **you, are in charge.** Believe me, it works. You will find that eventually you will have progressed so far you automatically abhor the cravings you could not say "no" to not so long ago. What is even more important, the decision is usually permanent. Your mind has accepted it, and will not question your authority.

At this stage, it is possible to change any habit, no matter how small or big. It is all a matter of application and perseverance. The process is so powerful that even the things that are strong in the line of enjoyment, especially those that you know are not to your benefit and are irresistible to you now, will become absolutely abhorrent should you choose it to be so. It becomes easier all the time.

Look forward to the stage where you will be in control to the extent that the hustle and bustle of this world will have no influence on or interrupt your thinking. *Make this chapter your constant companion, read it again and again until it becomes part of you. I suggest you read a piece every night before going to sleep. The last thoughts of the day are the ones our minds are more inclined to remember.*

Finally the soul... the soul is all emotion. This is where the finer, deeper and more powerful sides of a person are displayed. When a person's mind and soul combines, great philosophies on many subjects are possible A few examples are religion, the arts, poetry, etc. Good luck.

Chapter 12

DISCIPLINE

DISCIPLINE – HAPPINESS.

It is important to read the chapter on the mind first, before indulging in some more delicious reading on a subject that is closely related to the mind, as it will make this chapter a lot clearer and easier to understand.

What does "Never be bored again" sound like? Yes, it is quite possible to enjoy that particular mind control capacity by educating the mind with minimal effort.

The mind is bored simply because it is inactive. It is not designed to be in that particular mode; in other words, it is wondering. Once it has been educated to remain in positive mode it will stop wondering and think positive productive thoughts automatically. Completely effortless, all that is required is a little time and effort. *That is when the mind attracts ideas that are on the prowl looking for fertile ground.*

Attitude, a tool that is on average usually in automatic drive. Taken out of automatic, it becomes a mighty weapon that will with a little positive imagination and effort guide the operator towards huge successes he/she never thought possible.

Attitude is at the disposal of the person and not the mind, as is so often erroneously assumed. Yes, you, the person, can decide what kind of attitude will rule your life. It is as simple as that. Read on to see how that powerful force can become a reality in your life.

Wrong attitude or no attitude at all is due to negative or wrong belief, or no belief at all. This situation will be corrected by replacing the negative mindset with a positive one.

Without a positive and disciplined mind, it is impossible to achieve any measure of success. It is easily noticeable when the lack of discipline is widely present due to the evidence of lack of success, be it universal, in businesses or with individuals. Where success is present, discipline is the mainstay of success.

To be successful at a holistic way of life, a fair amount of discipline is necessary. If one is not a disciplined person it is not difficult to overcome the problem. All that is required is a little effort and know-how, a matter of changing your attitude to a positive and *progress* oriented one, a matter of learning and application, one small step at a time.

Before all this can take place it is important to know what causes the lack of discipline. Hopefully reading this will grab your attention and you will do a bit of soul-searching to fulfill your part of the bargain. It could be the most important revelation of your entire life. This recipe or principle to achieve success must be combined with the method described in the chapter on the mind, where we learned that the mind is easily manipulated. Right now any problem viewed at face value seems frightening and the prospect of solving it a daunting task. Following the principles described in the chapter on mind dynamics will help to solve the problem a whole lot easier, one tiny conscious effort at a time.

Now to see what the soul searching is all about. It may seem a bit unfair to ask an individual to perform self-analysis without psychological or professional help. This is also not a huge problem. Total self-honesty without delusion is all that is required.

It will soon become abundantly clear that many of the problems related to discipline or the lack thereof are, to name but a few: We think that other people are responsible for our well-being; we have no duties to perform to achieve success or satisfy our needs; we have no responsibility towards society; and perhaps one more very important one, "we are not responsible for our own failures."

Many people who have had an easy ride through life may not be aware, or will not know that their lack of progress is due to the fact that they were raised without the necessary restraint and guidance to instill a sense of discipline to ensure that they will one day be responsible adults. Should any of these suggestions prove to be insufficient, then it is abundantly clear that more in-depth psychological guidance is a dire necessity. This writing is by and large a "do it yourself" guide to success, and if success eludes you at the end of it, do make the effort to consult with a professional or some of the many books available on the subject. The end result will prove to be well worth the effort. You have the rest of your life ahead of you.

To consult with professionals carries no stigma whatsoever. It is merely to identify a deviation of one kind or another in the mind which needs to be corrected. One can relate it to any technical process that needs to be adjusted. It is human nature to assume that our problems are far worse than they really are and we are the only person to be so afflicted. To make an effort to solve your problems on your own, you have to be brutally honest with yourself and have a burning desire to improve upon your efforts to be successful in all aspects of your life. With a clear and open mind, think carefully where you fall short of the target and make a list. Apart from the few pointers listed above, there could many more, and that is not out of the ordinary. Provided you are totally honest, it will not be difficult to make a complete list no matter how unimportant and irrelevant an item may seem (you will be the only person who will have access to the list). They are all part of the same problem.

Select one of the areas in your life you would like to improve upon. To make things easy to understand, break the problem up into smaller sections by taking a hard look at that particular part of your life until you are convinced that you understand why things are not working out for you in that particular area. Carefully consider every aspect of the problem in the same way. Think in depth about what you have just discovered. Realise that things have to change. Think about the positive alternative with great care and always be objective. Hold onto that thought until your mind has accepted it as a reality and until it has become part of your mindset. Work through the whole problem, and when that has been completed you will notice a change within yourself. That is the beginning of successfully correcting your mindset.

Then move on to the next one, and the next. Before long you will feel elation at the success you are achieving. Stopping the process at this stage will not be an option for you. *Look at the whole process in a light-hearted manner. It does not have to weigh heavily on your mind. Have some fun while doing it. It may take some time before you realize what you are doing to improve your outlook on life is the most exciting and most wonderful exercise you have ever undertaken, and you can claim all the credit for your success. The sense of satisfaction will be enormous.*

Success is when your mind has accepted the change and it has become part of your personality. In other words, you are reprogramming not only your mind but the whole person. Do see it as a technical or practical rather than a psychological process. Believe that your mind is as average and normal as the next person.

Be positive that you will succeed in your efforts to bring about change. A positive mindset is of cardinal importance. If you feel you are not making progress, perhaps due to a lack of conviction as far as the method is concerned, do persist. Read it again, it deserves at least a second chance.

Success is not always achieved the first time around. It costs nothing apart from a little effort to do it without any thought of doubt or failure on your part, be positive at all times. Once you have given the process a fair chance without any success, then it is time to move on to perhaps more sophisticated help.

This method can work with many other social "problems" as well, which are usually attitudinal, attitude towards colleagues, work, or social relationships. These "problems" can have a more deep-seated origin. This method may be sufficient to achieve success. It may be worth the effort and go a long way towards changing your attitude towards people and see them in a more realistic and eventually a more positive light. This will put you in a more positive frame of mind and so boost your confidence. One of the most rewarding aspects of this method is the fact that you will learn to develop a more realistic attitude towards yourself. It will teach you to think rationally in general. You will soon find that you are far more able to do things on your own and do not have to rely on other people's advice, opinions, or approval.

Lack of confidence is more often than not at the root of poor discipline. For instance, deliberately being late for meetings and appointments is the worst example of being rude, although the offender does not see it as such because making a point of being noticed is of prime importance. The audience sees it for what it really is — a lack of discipline. Imagine what it does to the morale of the speaker who is all pumped up with nerves at breaking point.

Emotional problems. These we can add to the many books already written. This is a problem that touches every person on earth sometime during his/her lifetime. In the main, we will leave this one to the experts. Where it has not yet reached a level where professional help is needed, the method mentioned above may just be enough to avoid such a move. Nothing stops the individual from making a second or even a third effort at helping him or herself via this method to improve relationships with other people, be it social, work, sport, anywhere contact with people happens.

Problematic relationships are in the main created by parties not understanding one another, most often through sheer pride and stubbornness, refusing to see the other's point of view due to a lack of confidence and discipline within themselves. In their minds, they are already convinced they are right and the other is to blame. With such a short-sighted and narrow attitude, there will be no solution to any problem.

Hopefully, at least one party in a relationship will read this together with the chapter on how to create a positive mindset and realise that it is not difficult for someone with a confident mind to get on with another person without losing face if they make an effort to understand these very elementary principles, and realise that it is possible for a lay person to learn about and understand the basic principles of a relationship. Hope never despairs, as long as interest and willingness are in the offing and one is willing to grab the opportunity with both hands to better oneself. All that is required is to consider all the aspects of the problem thoroughly, realize where the obstacle lies, relinquish pride, and employ the thinking process. We do not live in an ideal world where success is always handed to us on a platter. We have to make some effort. The route to success is always via a well-disciplined mind.

Physical – here sport comes to mind immediately. Confidence is usually at the heart of the problem *Can* I do it? Can l achieve my goal, whatever? Do not compare yourself to others for we are not all at the same level. It is not winning all the time that matters, it is taking part that is important. To understand this statement, you must become aware of the fact that one always competes against oneself first, as long as there is **progress**. Once you realize and understand that, you will feel liberated. Use the method to build confidence. Once you have done that, you will be in a much better frame of mind to decide whether you will make the grade or not, and can consider at what level you could successfully compete with other people, should that be important to you. The choice remains yours.

After reading the chapter on the mind and gaining a lot more confidence, it will not matter whether you win or lose. Winning is important simply because it is nice to win, but from now on it will be no big deal if you do not win. The difference in attitude will bring about an enormous change in your personality. It will touch every aspect of your person, you will see people (and yourself) in a different light and other people will look at you differently, in a more positive way. You will certainly feel the difference, and to you, the sky is the limit to what level of success you will achieve. All that can come about with a simple change of attitude. Then you will feel like and be a winner.

In this particular way, lives can be turned around and changed for the better. For instance, a confused and wondering mind can become a disciplined and organized one. Negative thoughts are a very powerful force, they have the ability to feed on one another and become most destructive.

Some unfortunate people go through their entire life locked into this disadvantaged frame of mind, not knowing that it is possible to change. Even emotional problems, spawned by constant negative thinking that has escalated out of control, can still result in a changed life after applying this process, combined with the one described in the chapter on the mind. Be on your guard, these little blighters should be nipped in the butt as soon as they are noticed, which should be much easier from now on.

Thinking in the negative constantly, you have very little chance of becoming successful at anything. Negative folk seldom achieve much. The motivation is just not there. They seldom make an attempt at anything that requires a reasonable amount of effort and are usually defeated prematurely, even during the process of conceiving an idea. Because they have no self-confidence, their mind, which as a matter of course is constantly immersed in a sea of negativity, automatically rejects the idea that could very well have been a winner. Another opportunity lost – had they dug just a little further they may very well have struck gold.

The effort seems too big, too awesome. The inferior image they have created of themselves, or perhaps were forced upon them through unavoidable circumstances such as an unfortunate childhood, convinced them that they are not capable of achieving any success in life. Due to no fault of their own, they are unwittingly locked into a negative frame of mind. This can all be changed as they usually fall within the average person category.

By applying the principles mentioned above, one small step at a time, success is inevitable. Such people need to be convinced they have to make an effort to take that first step. Often just a small success story is enough to turn a situation around, and you already have the beginning of a changed mind and a changed person with new prospects, a new life, and much to look forward to. The average person is capable of great success, if only he can realize and understand that his conceived dreams are possible and he can make them happen.

Nobody is immune to the feeling of delight when success has finally been achieved. Success is for everybody with enthusiasm, not only brilliant minds.

Somewhere inside all of us, at some time or another, there is a desire to achieve, to create, to build, make or manufacture. That desire needs to be nurtured, even if it seems an impossible task. The bigger the problem, the sweeter the success. Don't look at the problem head on, study the project in detail, pull it apart, dissect it, concentrate on one detail at a time. Then decide what you will attempt first. All you need is your first success. The flame will be lit and will grow bigger and stronger and what do we have? – another changed life!

See it as fun and not as a huge mountain to climb, figuratively speaking. Once you have your first success in the bag you will never be able to stop, so start small.

Solving problems, climbing mountains, achieving success is great fun, whether it is work or play. Enjoy yourself, see things in a light-hearted way. So what if you fail? That should be the essence of your life. Your first success will be your greatest triumph.

There are many different reasons why people lack confidence or live in a negative world and are consequently deprived of success and happiness. There are always answers to their problems. If they are deep-seated, a professional person can usually offer help and one should not hesitate to approach such a person. As mentioned before, in the past there was a stigma attached to the idea of seeking help on the mental or emotional level. Thankfully, those nonsensical notions have been done away with. There has hardly been any great person during this modern era who has reached great heights, and not been under incredible stress sometime during his/her lifetime, and has not asked for help from a professional. Many big corporations have such professionals on their payroll.

Counseling is an accepted practice in the modern era the world over. Professional counselors receive counseling after every complicated case they were involved with. It is just a state of mind that has to be corrected, and the way the professional does it is one small step at a time. Success, happiness, and joy, should be part of everybody's life.

Now to bolster and build upon the success you have achieved and move on to the next step. Concentrate on all the positive aspects of your life. Take your time and make a list of anything positive that has happened, any success you were responsible for, no matter how small and insignificant they may seem. Concentrate on them and visualize them growing in stature until you see their very important intrinsic value, and the role they play in your life.

Now use that ammunition together with what you have learned from the chapter on mind control. Remember it is all about thinking, positive thinking, see the wood from the trees, no more negative thinking, all positive. Remember ***positive thoughts attract positive thoughts. Consequently, a positive mind attracts positive minds.*** That way you grow in stature and importance. Do not stop doing this until you look in the mirror and see that very significant different look in your eyes.

The eyes are the windows of the soul. When you have progressed enough you will be able to look into another person's eyes and gauge his level of confidence, and later on, even what he thinks. Then you will know that you have achieved a gigantic level of success and growth. Other people will notice it and treat you differently. Remember, all it takes is effort. You are more than likely within the average category, just like many of us.

When you look in the mirror and the confidence shows in your eyes, you will realise you are beginning to see the light and get the feeling that you are on the brink of understanding what the saying, *you know that you know that you know* is all about, and you will be able to achieve all that your mind can believe you can achieve, probably the greatest revelation you will ever experience, a light bulb moment! Probably more like a lightning strike! Yes, it can happen to you, no matter who you are. To substantiate and understand this statement, one must realize that at any time we use only a fraction of our brain power, there is plenty left for further use. You are no less capable of achieving success than any other person of average capability. (Make the highlighted statement above a mantra to carry with you wherever you go).

It is often said that doting mothers are their son's worst enemies, and when the son is academically gifted it can be a disaster of major proportions for the unfortunate fellow. The mother is over-protective, unwittingly the son learns and becomes conditioned early in life that he can get away with whatever he chooses to, he does not have to lift a finger to help with chores around the house. The chores are all done for him. The father sees what the situation is leading to, has from experience learned not to interfere, and against his better judgment and for the sake of peace or saving feelings from being hurt, simply lets it slide and hopes for the best.

Come Varsity, he usually does not have to put in much effort to achieve success. Usually the best employment finds him, rather than the other way around. What you learn during childhood stays with you throughout your entire life, unless you are fortunate enough to have learned via writings such as these that it can be changed.

Unfortunately, the opposite is also true, the lack of what you should have learned, but have not, also stays with you. This person has never learned to cooperate or share with other children or family members at home.

Now at Varsity he discovers there are certain parameters that have to be respected but does not know why or how it is done. Soon he finds himself very unpopular with not only his fellow students and superiors, but later co-workers as well. What is his home life like? More than likely very much in the same vein?

In the event you recognize yourself and would like to be successful, decide to make a change to your attitude. After all, you are of superior enough intelligence.

Unless the gifted child has learned from an early age the intricacies of discipline, cooperation, and that life is not one big bowl of cherries, that there are challenges to be met and overcome to prepare oneself for the rigors of life, he will find it tough out there. There are many reasons why the failure rate is so high amongst students from the higher echelons of education, professionals who sit behind desks shuffling papers, selling insurance or investments. (Not that there is anything wrong with selling of any kind. l have done that kind of work for many years, and will gladly admit that l enjoyed it enormously, found it very rewarding both financially and otherwise. It supplied me with an education where l learned an enormous amount about the human psyche. Volunteering for the door-to-door form of marketing provided me with the opportunity to enter so many homes and to learn so much about people, their personalities, and how they live, one place where everybody is himself. (Knowledge gained that is part of me and I will not trade it for the world). Surely that is not what these professionals originally imagined, expected or envisaged for themselves.

My interest in human behavior exposed me to an enormous number of qualified individuals who were academically gifted but never rose above the level of mediocrity. It is absolutely possible for them to become intellectuals as well and then the sky is the limit towards achieving success, for instance developing their thinking ability with the help of mind dynamics, i.e. *progressive* positive thinking, if only they could realize that.

One reason for the substantial failure rate is quite easy to understand. The gifted academic who was blessed with a retentive memory never found it difficult to study, he would read and remember. Come exam time he or she would disgorge the information with minimal effort compared to his/her counterpart who had to study, think, and apply him or herself. The constant application of faculties, thought and thinking, exercised their thinking ability of the latter. That developed the intellectual side of their brain. It is not possible to achieve success without extensive use and training of the intellectual abilities. It may not be easy, but it will be necessary to develop and use specialized thinking. The current mold will have to be broken and the new one needs to be discovered and developed.

Life is not always unfair, as we so often like to believe when we compare ourselves to these "fortunate" people. Much better to go through life as an average person where discipline is the order of the day. It exposes a person to training through experience that would otherwise not have been the case. Every experience is a small part of a learning curve, and it is important to see it as such. This automatically expands one's thinking ability, teaches one to cooperate, enhances one's social standing in society and sporting activities, and enables one to learn what teamwork is all about, which leads to feelings of satisfaction that are so important in creating positive feelings and an attitude that leads to eventual success.

Those of us who did not have it as "good" as the first mentioned, who had to fight for every bit of progress under what seemed to be very unfair circumstances and at a great disadvantage, are probably right. Life did treat them unfairly, but you can still be a winner, and to you winning will mean so much more. Hardship builds character. You have trained your mind, expanded your thinking ability, learned how to use your imagination, and all will come together to defeat those feelings of being hard done by. In the end, your sense of achievement will be so much sweeter and you will be so much richer in experience. Remember, for every measure of hardship, there is an equal or larger measure of positive outcome. In the end, you win every time.

Now you can move on the same level or even surpass your peers. It is a fact that work creates a sense of joy, and success a sense of achievement. Your life will be so much happier and if not better, at least a lot sweeter. You have achieved so much more; you have done it. Will you not be proud of yourself? You did it on your own, all by yourself. You did not have the unseen support the gifted person had. Satisfaction is so much greater. It often crosses my mind that the life of a gifted person sometimes seems to be a humdrum affair. *After all, an enormous amount of joy and happiness is derived through the effort to achieve eventual success.*

Like the good Book says, "give thanks in all things." You are a winner more than likely because of the fact that you had to make a bigger effort. Consequently, you have also won bigger, where it matters – in the mind. Experiences are the wealth of life, *not always money*. How I often pity the "money at all cost" attitude, they miss out on so much in life where real happiness is to be found. *We only live once, and it is how we fill the period between from the beginning to the end that matters, not how much you accumulate materially.*

The essence of life is made up of what you experience with *a positive attitude.* Every incident, *good or bad,* will have a positive spin-off. You learn from both, and it adds to the enrichment of the mind when it will stand you in good stead later in life. You know so much more than the person who has had a magic carpet ride through life.

You not only know theoretically what hardship is, you have felt it, experienced it, your mind is crammed full of events that happened to you or around you. They may have been unpleasant and negative at the time but they have all added to your wealth of knowledge, **enriching your mind.**

You have seen how the other side lives. You have experienced what other people have only read about or learned about second-hand. They will never know what it is like to experience it first-hand, whereas you do. Knowledge is always power. Do not for one moment allow these chapters in your life to hamper your progress. Remember you are the one who owns the degree earned at the University of Life. Take advantage of the situation, you are so much stronger than the "fortunate" ones. If I had it easy during my early life on this earth, there is no way that I would be able to write what I am writing now, and hopefully influence others in a positive way.

If they benefit and become successful, then the effort on my part will have been worthwhile and I will be eternally grateful for having had the opportunity to be involved. I would not change places with the first mentioned for all the material riches in the world. *Every experience, good or bad is a positive one, you learn from bot. Money is not the measure of success. Success is the sum total of what you have experienced, and the successes you have achieved*

are the riches form of reward. This is what is of lasting value, what fills the mind and consumes the imagination. In later years, this will be the driving force to a happy and contented life. Those are the times when one lives off memories, the more the richer, the sweeter the better.

The University of Life is nothing to be ashamed of and everything to be proud of. There you will find an enormous amount of positivity, emanating from your experiences. You will never suffer from tunnel vision as is the case of so many people who have achieved degrees. So often they have, without being aware of it, adopted the attitude, *Now, I am educated and know it all.* Life is never that easy, it is one long study session and one never knows it all. Should you be tempted to think this way be careful, you may eventually end up in a place of discontent and be a monumental bore. Remember, you were educated in only one direction to make you an expert in that particular field, there are many more.

At the University of Life, you have to put in so much more effort to educate yourself. You are obliged to cover so much more territory, consequently, you know about so many different angles life presents you with. Allow me to say, success is relevant, like all things in life, to the amount of effort you are prepared to muster. By now that should not be a problem, provided you have taken to heart what you have read and even done some experimenting. Your curiosity has been stirred and you cannot wait to see what there is waiting for you around the next corner.

Most people would like to have enjoyed the benefit of a good education. Unfortunately, that is just not possible for all. Success is possible for those who persevere.

Education is not the panacea in life as it is sometimes made out to be. It is not the only route and is not essential to achieve success, provided you are willing to learn and apply yourself. Here is where you can learn how to do it. **If you can read, you can educate yourself.**

Not for a moment do I want to denigrate education. That goes without saying. I am merely pointing out there are alternatives to formal education for the less fortunate ones who never had the privilege to enter through the hallowed portals of a University. Chasing money and making it your sole purpose in life certainly has merit, especially for those who enjoy doing just that. However, it consumes so much time and energy that could have been spent on more worthwhile matters, that will have much more intrinsic value in the long run when we realize that financial wealth is not all that it is made out to be and that the *mind and its related doings are of far higher value.*

Chapter 13

ENTREPRENEURS

We are not yet done with the mind and related matters. Entrepreneurial concerns also begin and end in the mind. This is the practical side and expression of what is conceived in the mind.

To be an entrepreneur is a way of life and I do think to be successful at it, it would be advisable to study the previous two chapters which will make it so much easier to understand an already complicated career choice. This is not my first, no, it is my only choice, to make a living and also not only to make a living, it is the only way of life for me. It is rough, it is tough, it is hard and that is the way I like it. The eventual success is so sweet.

Having read the previous two chapters, it should be clear why I derive so much pleasure from the workings of the mind. Entrepreneurial matters are just another extension thereof and success will be so much easier to achieve once the principle is understood.

In this chapter we will continue to weave the two together until it becomes clear how an entrepreneur is born. To be an entrepreneur is to be successful in many directions. It becomes a way of life, you become success minded, success in any direction you choose and not only in the "megabucks" category. Only a very small percentage of the money-chasing wannabes ever make it to be successful in the big league. That means you will not be stranded if you do not make it "big," but you will have an enormous amount of knowledge to fall back on with the entrepreneurial spirit on your side.

The failure rate of success in the big league is enormous, more often than not with dire consequences for themselves and their families. So much time is wasted and often it is too late to make a change for the better, which is usually the one that would have made more sense right from the beginning, but is usually too mundane to satisfy their ambition. Is it worth the effort and energy spent on the mad chase to achieve "big" financial success? A life with a "multi-dimensionally developed mind," is definitely the better choice.

A success-oriented mind will be of great benefit in whatever direction you choose. For instance, would it not be a better choice to be financially secure in good employment with a good pension plan, and to make sure there is enough time to spend on matters concerning the mind, body, and soul of not only yourself but the family, where all joy and happiness is registered, where the real riches lie? I cannot but wonder when talking with these "mighty" men who have made it in their "real" world, one can almost read their minds when they wonder: *is this all there is to it? I expected so much more.* I am not impressed, and not surprised so many "successful" people have found in the end their family and private lives are anything but successful. Perhaps they have put in so much time and effort to achieve their dream, they have missed out on the really important matters concerning life, and also the smaller irritations that make life a worthy cause.

Think clearly and with a sober mind what negative aspects affect the lives of the famous and the very wealthy. It is not all positive. Fame and fortune have a huge negative side as well. The moment you become famous you lose your personal freedom, you become public property. Out the window fly all the little things you used to enjoy and took for granted, like enjoying an uninterrupted meal in a restaurant without at best being noticed, or at worst being swamped by adoring fans. Or a peaceful, leisurely walk on the beachfront. Losing all that is not my idea of a good life. There are without question many people who would love that to happen to them, but if you are a person who enjoys your privacy and likes the simple things in life, then that kind of "good fortune" would be like a millstone around your neck.

Should you decide to go the entrepreneurial route, do so by all means. You may find the following few snippets useful along the way.

Be careful which way to go when you decide to take the independent route. Consider all your options, weigh up the one against the other, write the pros and cons down on paper, do not leave out any detail no matter how unimportant it may seem, and then make a decision. Until you are a well-seasoned entrepreneur, speak to experts in a field related to the one you are interested in. We always look at our own ideas through rose-coloured glasses. The fact it is your idea does so much for the ego it tends to cloud all sense of reality, so ask what other people think. Make sure you ask successful people for their opinion. Discussing your project with someone who knows only as much as, or even less than you do, on the subject because you don't have the courage to ask successful people, is not a good idea, I found successful people of good character usually willing to part with good advice, as long as it does not clash with their own strategies and interest. They have been through the mill. Be sure of the kind of questions, as well as all your facts and figures, before you approach them.

Several aspiring tycoons have approached me over the years on account of the fact that I have been successful at marketing. They always had an article they had gone to great length and expense to develop. It usually involved plastic injection molding, a very expensive process which takes an enormous amount of time, and time is money. Unfortunately, everyone was of such a nature that it would have been impossible to achieve any measure of success. The negative answer was usually not only my own, but that of other persons well versed in business matters I approached for a second opinion. It is not a pleasant task to burst someone's bubble, his dream, and hope of success. To soften the blow, my answer was always to ask for more opinions. If only they had asked for advice before entering uncharted waters because some of the deals involved large sums of money.

The road to success is not an easy one, but well worth the effort, I do not for one moment knock entrepreneurship. That is how 1 made a living for most of my adult life, not always successfully but on average far more plusses than negatives. Just believe that you can do it; you can acquire the necessary knowledge. What you are reading now is your textbook to achieving success. Remember it is yours, you have earned it and it is so sweet; the satisfaction is worth every effort.

Being an entrepreneur is not for the faint-hearted. It is hard to compete with hard-nosed businessmen and women. Sometimes you wonder how many more punches you can endure. Then, just when you think you have reached the end of your tether, the tide always turns when the right moment arrives. In this world nothing is for nothing and very little for something, but that something is always worth the effort. Although it may not seem so, there are more plus sides to the story than negative ones, and success is so sweet, apart from the fact that, in addition, it provides a lot of excitement during one's working career.

You have to wear so many different hats – the manager, the psychologist, counselor, salesman, and so many more. You have to be competent at all of them, else you will not succeed, if any one of them lacks. Don't be discouraged you will learn rapidly from your mistakes.

For instance, marketing – you can own the largest warehouse in the world filled to the brim, but if you cannot shift the goods they are totally worthless to you. Next time, when derogatory thoughts concerning salesmen pass through your mind, think again. A good marketing man is the key that will unlock the door to Aladdin's cave. It is essential that you as the principal in the enterprise become proficient at marketing. Even if it means you have to gain some direct experience at some form of marketing, it is advisable you embark on this road before you start a business.

Start slowly and learn as you go along. Far too often someone by chance comes into a lot of money, and without experience starts a business that overwhelms him and ends in disaster. The subsequent knock may be so severe that, sadly, he may never attempt another venture, when it could have been an exciting and successful life. I have personally had several experiences where an individual asked for advice, did not follow the given advice, and subsequently failed.

Learn in a small way, and slowly, if you do not have the "know how" and experience to help you make a success of your venture. So often we hear the remark, "I want to start my own business" or "I have started a business," from someone with absolutely no experience in business matters.

It is far too often assumed one is born with the gift of experience or business "know how." It is arguably the most difficult step one can take in life and also the most important. Don't forget our more fortunate brothers and sisters who had the advantage of learning at the Varsity, or perhaps gained experience via an established family business.

However, don't despair, you can do it. Just be careful and be wide awake.

A rash and reckless move could turn out to be the person's nemesis, with serious consequences not only for himself but people he is connected with. It is so important, allow me to repeat, it is better to start small and gain experience. Even if you have sufficient funds tread carefully, it could save a lot of those valuable funds in the long run.

There is a similarity to all professions, the same as with technical work. You have to serve an "apprenticeship" and learn the "know how" of the particular business you intend to enter into. Whether big or small makes no difference, but the smaller the better with much less risk, until you are familiar with business know-how.

Be particularly careful when the intention is to buy a business. The minefields are many and enormous, especially in the case of a small business. There are always reasons why the business is for sale, and the given one is seldom the honest one. Unless you are in that specific kind of business and know it inside out, as well as the running of it, spend some money on professional guidance to help you to decide. It may be expensive, but cheaper in the long run.

A very common way the less than honest broker, usually very experienced and a smooth operator, sells a business to a victim is by finding someone who he can see, on account of past experience, will not make the grade.

He will approach the intended victim, usually a young and inexperienced candidate, and sell the business to him with lots of smooth tal, on the never, never system, usually with a large upfront payment and monthly installments he knows the buyer will not be able to afford. The unsuspecting victim is made to believe the unrealistic terms are easily manageable. There usually is a clause included in the contract stating if one or perhaps two monthly payments have been missed the ownership of the business reverts back to the seller. These clauses are usually well disguised in legal jargon.

Businesses like these are usually sold many times over. The victims have no comeback for the villain has legally done nothing wrong. Even the legal costs will be for the account of the victim. This is a very common ploy. I personally had first-hand experience where the same motor vehicles were sold over and over up to five times to different eager owners. I worked for the company for only a short while, until I became aware of the dishonesty.

While entrepreneurship is still the only way for many of us to go and is the backbone of any country's economy (it employs vast numbers of people), and a very exciting way to live, the previous example must be taken seriously. It is very tempting for the ambitious young person who desperately wants to be his/her own boss to say no to such an attractive deal that has been so carefully prepared. You have to have the proverbial hair on your teeth and be very tough when you negotiate. Do not be afraid to ask penetrating questions, and don't lose your nerve when the perpetrator threatens to withdraw his offer by saying you will never again be offered such an opportunity. Should that be the case he is more than likely sensing you are wide awake. This is the time to disagree and forget about the fortune he promised you would lose should your answer be no.

Large amounts of money are seldom the vehicle to happiness. There are many conditions that have to be met to ensure a happy and contented life. Staring yourself blind at the prospect of making big money as the be all and end all to happiness is downright foolish and short sighted. Money is low down on the list of whatever it takes to bring happiness, as the following story will tell. And if that is not the case, then hopefully after reading this you will come to better insight and are a much wiser person.

Personal experiences usually speak volumes. The following has always weighed heavily on my mind and I feel compelled to mention it. It is about the son of one of the big industrialists in the country living next door to me. He was in his early twenties, very pleasant, but also lonely and sad in spite of having a young lady in his life and obviously enough money. There was an instinctive reason for me to befriend this young man and I subsequently got to know a fair amount about his private life. He received a healthy allowance, plus a free apartment, as well as a motor vehicle. He was well cared for materially, but emotionally sadly neglected. Over the years I knew him I was not aware of any family member paying him a visit.

Many years later, although I had never met his parents, by chance because of the unusual surname, I discovered I was talking with his mother. I had grown fond of the young man and wanted to know how he was getting on. What a shock it was to hear he had taken his own life. I did not know all the details of this sad and lonely young man's life, and nobody has the right to judge. Nevertheless, the impression it left with me was a very sad one.

Not all fortune-seekers shirk their responsibilities towards their families. Society is teeming with wonderful examples of people who come from wealthy backgrounds who obviously had great parents with high social standing and integrity. Consequently, they in turn became successful parents with happy family lives.

We cannot do without these captains of industry. They supply the life support in the form of jobs and cause the economy to grow. That does not mean you have to feel it is the only way to success and happiness in life. There are many different ways to success, and if need be, change your perception to a more realistic one. Be your own person, you don't have to be one of them.

The well-balanced human mind that is not only concerned with material things, will provide satisfaction in both the emotional, mental, and eventually the material side as well, the engine room of life where problems are solved and ideas are born, where anything material is low down on the list of priorities. That is where real growth takes place, where you become an emotional millionaire, and the taste is just as sweet, if not more so.

If you follow the example of successful graduates from the University of Life, you will be a winner on account of the wider outlook on life you were forced to experience, and eventually be financially secure and successful. Instead of staring yourself blind at the mere prospect of having a lot of money, by following directions where other matters that are not money-related and equally or even more important, you will gain much experience that will make it easier to be financially successful. The number of directions you can follow is enormous. On account of your having experienced so much more during your sometimes turbulent life, it is so much easier to spot the different opportunities when they do come your way. Do not be desperate. Think clearly, there is hope for everybody, including you.

Thomas Edison, one of the greatest inventors the world ever saw, made so many attempts at the electric light bulb that he lost count and although it took him years to perfect it, he never gave up. Imagine if he did! Never give up, after digging for miles you may be just one meter away from the gold reef you are looking for. If you give up, someone else may come along and complete the digging.

We all have heard of stepping stones. Don't despair, remember *"when the going gets tough the tough gets going."* Use every stone as a step up to the next one and learn from everyone you leave behind. Gaining knowledge is never a waste of time even if it seems so; you may have a need for it at a later stage. It is not how many times you fall down, it is how many times you get up and continue.

Learn to think outside the box. Think past barriers and parameters. Do not accept you are not allowed to, or not capable of operating outside those boundaries.

A word of advice for prospective entrepreneurs: So much time and energy is spent on trying to find the elusive new idea that will bring the proverbial fortune within reach. There are seven billion people on earth and it seems almost everyone is looking for the missing charm that will be their golden nugget. It is like taking a lottery ticket. A lottery ticket is equated to an ocean with one fish in it and fifty million people with fishing rods hoping to be the lucky one to catch the fish. There are those who were successful, but unfortunately, the odds stacked against you are enormous. So rather spend all that valuable time and energy on a more realistic way to success. Start making your own success, now that you are beginning to learn how to.

The danger of getting hooked on being the fortunate one to win the elusive prize in a lottery is a dangerous game to play. You are slowly being dragged into the flights of fantasy week after week, until it becomes a pattern from which it will be very difficult to dislodge yourself. A slippery slope is more often than not a sure destination for those unfortunate folk.

The best advice any business man can pass on to you will be to *"find a need and fill it."* It is not easy, but a lot more realistic. Needs appear everywhere, all the time. Changes and improvements are taking place so fast it is almost impossible to keep pace. With the knowledge you have acquired by studying the chapter on the mind, it will be much easier for you to spot the opportunities. To make changes or improvements to any object that carries a patent can, within reason and after careful consideration of legal implications, be changed and be registered.

Patent rights are flouted continuously and there are many ways to get away with it scot free. To register a patent worldwide, it has to be registered in every country individually where it can possibly be manufactured. That makes the process impossible except for the financially well-healed. Forget about patents, it is a complicated and very expensive process and most of the time not worth the effort. Someone in a country so small you may never have heard of, and which has missed the patent holder's attention, with a few minor changes to the design and some sound legal advice can go right ahead and produce the product without fear of prosecution.

Apparently, there are more inventions sitting in drawers that have not been registered. Try and find improvements that can be turned into viable propositions. Take note of the age-old and still the most successful advice mentioned above in bold letters.

Be proactive. Through positive thinking, develop your initiative by being bold and learn to see opportunities where other people cannot. Allow your mind free rein, wherever you come into contact with any business establishment See if there is some way they are doing something you could do better or faster, or in a slightly different way. This is an art form, once developed can be very profitable. I have done it several times. Keep looking until you become proficient at the art of spotting an opportunity. Eventually, you will be doing this every waking moment of the day. It makes life very interesting and kills boredom.

Never forget that work is a privilege, and not a right. God has designed it in that particular way not only to make life more interesting, it is essential to maintain discipline. To sit around all day wishing time away is the most destructive condition we can bring upon ourselves. Nothing can beat the feeling of fulfillment when a piece of work is brought to a satisfactory conclusion. And for entrepreneurs, there is the added joy of knowing you have initiated it all and it is your creation. When we understand and perhaps have experienced that joy, then it is easy to see how such a person can turn into a workaholic.

In most countries, the government makes assistance available to talented people who can turn good ideas into profit. By now you have learned how to spot opportunities. Expose yourself to every bit of information from every quarter you can think of until your brain triggers off a possibility. It will take a lot of brainwork and effort, but by now you will know how much joy can be had from using the gray matter. The subsequent success will always be far greater than any effort you will make.

You may be of the opinion that you simply cannot do it. However, you will never know until you have made an attempt at doing something that simply seems too big and unattainable for you to manage. Don't sell yourself short, investigate all prospects thoroughly, never give up until you are totally convinced it is simply not possible for you to manage such a project. You will never know until you have tried and you may surprise yourself. Man's ingenuity must not be underestimated, and that includes yours as well. Remember, do not wait for it to happen, **make it happen. Don't wait for it to come to you, go and fetch it. Nothing happens without effort. By doing a lot will gain you a lot, doing something will gain you something, doing nothing will gain you nothing.**

Never think of yourself as "ordinary." **Nothing** ordinary has ever excelled beyond or above the ordinary, and our mind is certainly not a thing. It is our most prized possession and needs to be respected as such. **Aim for the moon and you will hit the rooftops. Be realistic but not conservative when you set your targets. You will be aiming at many more targets than you have done in the past, and will not reach every single one, but will for certain be successful many more times than you were in the past. That way you will be sure to enjoy the success you should be dreaming of at this stage of your life.**

Take care not to allow money to become the overriding factor when you first think of starting your business. It is not the most important factor in this equation. Perseverance, knowledge on the subject, knowledge of human nature and behavior, research, and most of all, the passion and will to succeed is what will carry you to success. When you have met all these needs, money has a habit of appearing without much effort.

Working from home, if at all possible, is one way to reduce cost. The cost of rented accommodation is a huge drag on the finances (and profits) of any small business. That means that you will be able to charge the Receiver of Revenue a discount on your tax bill for space occupied by your business, and you score twice.

Signing a rental agreement always leaves one with a hollow feeling in the stomach, so work from home if at all possible, or a small rented property available on a monthly basis in a residential area. Many businesses were born in kitchens. I have been guilty of that on more than one occasion. This is where you can do all the experimenting that needs to be done. Something that cannot be emphasized enough, do not look at your intended effort through rose-coloured glasses. Be realistic do not allow your ambition to override your common sense.

The Far East has scored handsomely by following the same route when they were building their world, dominating enterprises by allowing their people (not employees, they are now self-employed), to work at their homes. For instance, manufacturing small parts for a larger end product that is put together in a much smaller factory than would otherwise be the case had the whole process taken place under one roof. Often the mother business would even supply the machines needed to do the work. This can often involve a large number of workers. Everyone scores, the mother factory saves on floor space, no involvement with unions, and administration staff is at a minimum.

The worker is now an entrepreneur, no longer an employee. He is proud of his new-found status and the quality of his products are much better. He works much longer hours, something he may have had to do in the past with a feeling of resentment, now is sheer pleasure. Quality control by the mother company is much easier. The actual physical cost can be lower on account of the self-motivation of the workers and saving on expensive floor space and a whole lot of other expenses, mean overheads are a fraction of what they would otherwise have been, resulting in cheaper products that can be delivered at an enormous cost advantage.

This way of doing the work is a great incentive for the workers. Most people cherish the idea of one day owning their own business or simply being self-employed. There is no more "clock" watching. They work at their own pace, often at an accelerated one. They keep their own hours, which are usually much longer. They don't have to go to and from work, and are with their families whenever it suits them. No more blue Mondays. All the days enjoy the same status, each one a joyful one, and most of all they earn far more than in a conventional way of employment.

Imagine this idea taking off in popularity all over the world. The enormous amount of fuel and energy saved, and global warming cut by large margins. Self-employment should be one of the main issues to be considered worldwide, especially where unemployment is a big headache to the authorities. Computers have brought about a veritable revolution in this respect which is growing at an enormous rate.

When all is said and done, there are also horses for courses. We don't always make the right choice the first time around. Don't despair – it happens every day somewhere in the world. It will be much easier for you to bring about a difference in attitude and change on account of the fact you did not have it easy, and the mind control you have learned and the wide variety of experiences you have gained during your learning period. Your staying powers have been tested so many times more than those who had it "easy." Keep a cool head, think it through carefully, weigh up the pros and cons and then decide. Don't waste time and energy on fantasies that will never work. Life has a way of rewarding people for sober and realistic efforts made, perhaps not the way or form in which you expected, but it will happen, probably when you least expect it.

Remember knowledge is power. Obtain it at every possible opportunity.

To live a full life, there must be a change in the outlook of the person who has a desire to succeed and, unfortunately, possesses a mind that is closed to ideas of any positive nature or creative ability. Remember no condition is permanent, np matter how many times you were told you would never make it. Provided you are not mentally deficient or impaired, you are as normal as any other person who was successful at something attempted. All that remains is for you to make the effort to remove the remaining imagined mental obstacles still holding you back. You and only you can do that. You have the necessary knowledge you have gained so far at your disposal should you want to refresh your memory. Make the effort now and put thoughts and words into action.

Chapter 14

SKIN AND SOAP

This will take most of you by surprise. I don't think I have many people who agree with my way of thinking, that is, except those of you who are on to the bandwagon that flies the holistic way of life flag and are aware of the effects soap has on the skin. Allow me to highlight some facts and win some converts to the wonderful world of having a skin made in heaven, soft as silk, free to function as a natural creation instead of being bullied and unjustly punished for being something it should not be – grimy and smelly. Then it can only be cleaned by the most barbaric means and measures imaginable, being scrubbed and washed with all kinds of cleaning materials meant for anything but the human skin, while all it is pleading for is to be cleaned with the most natural cleaning material on earth – water.

Generally speaking, the body is probably the least understood object we come in contact with every minute of every day and nothing more so than the skin, the, most misunderstood organ. We take the skin for granted, believing the skin is similar to a very versatile and tough plastic wrapper protecting us against the elements. No, it is a lot more than that. Let's have a closer look and pay a tribute to the skin, the most marvelous of organs and the biggest in the body.

It is only over the last decade or so science has managed to produce something that can perform some of the functions the skin is responsible for, but by far not as efficient as the skin and restricted to a few functions required by industry. It is alive and breathes, it allows moisture to escape and keeps outside what should remain outside, yet remains waterproof. It holds the body together, and is the first line of defense against the tremendous onslaught of the elements, among others.

The first thing we notice when we make visual contact with another person is the quality of their skin, usually a pleasant experience when it is a friend or someone we had not seen in a while. The reason people make so much effort caring for the skin on their face is surely to present themselves the best way possible. The cosmetic industry is one of the biggest and most powerful in the world, mainly directed at the appearance. None of them would think of offering natural holistic ways and means to achieve the results we see around us. At present the industry is far too lucrative. There is a more holistic and natural way to achieve the same results.

The body does not consist of a face alone, there is a whole lot more to it. The average person can't possibly treat the whole body in the same way the face is treated. To achieve the same results in a much more cost-effective way is there for everybody to enjoy. The answer is simply to ***stop washing with soap.***

Looking at the skin in more depth and really finding out what it is all about, what it consists of, and how it works is so awesome. It does become a little tedious when we discuss the body and mention again and again what a miraculous creation it is. Skin keeps moisture in and it keeps water out, and at the same time it breathes. The enormous role the skin plays in the total functioning of the body, and how integrated it is in the process, is demonstrated by the fact that if the skin for one reason or another is prevented from breathing we will suffocate and die. When all is not well within the body, the resultant condition is reflected on the skin. Even when we are emotionally overwrought, the skin is where it will be displayed for all to see. The skin is highly elastic and has enormous stretching ability. Let your mind wonder and think how it is possible to put on an enormous amount of weight and then lose it again, and within reason it returns to the original size and shape.

We perspire to keep cool, same as the radiator in a motor car or an air conditioner, allowing the moisture to escape, and as soon as the air passes over the skin the moisture evaporates and leaves us feeling cool. The skin also removes toxins from the body by allowing impurities to escape. Critics will be quick to point out that it is dirt, and the only way to rid the skin of these undesirables,, is to use soap. You could not do the skin a greater injustice. ***Everything that emanates from the*** *skin is water-soluble and is easily washed off with clean water only. No artificial cleaning materials are necessary.* Immediately external dirt comes to mind, so read on, this question will not remain a question for long. There is a more natural way to look after your skin, especially men, who usually do not like putting creams and the like on their skin, I for one can't tolerate creams, oils and lotions, rubbed or wiped all over me.

The skin, like every other organ in the body, is totally self-sufficient and takes care of its own maintenance. The skin consists of several layers, each with its own particular function. The epidermis is the one on the outside, and is by definition pretty robust, yet soft and smooth. It has to tolerate enormous abuse from every quarter, but still is only human tissue. The body cells, made from a combination of natural chemicals, are tough but only to the point that they are designed to handle natural cleaning materials like water that has been in existence for as long as skin has. Definitely not soap, which is laden with unnatural chemical cleaning agents. We do not need soap to clean ourselves. Water can do the job better than any artificial substitute, not only to clean ourselves but to achieve an amazing end result.

This may sound like a wild statement. Not really, there are many people who do not use soap, and have never used soap the superior quality of their skin is always the first to be noticed.

God made skin, He did not make soap. That was invented by man to wash clothing with and a very good idea, but not for the skin, so tender, yet so resilient. Soap, being a chemical not designed for the body, is totally incompatible with efforts to care for and look after the well-being of the skin. It dehydrates the skin and kills millions and millions of skin cells, and in the process the skin is robbed of its natural way to protect itself. To restore the skin is something man cannot do. Only the body can do that. Unfortunately, before the body can finish the task of rebuilding the cells, the process of destruction is repeated. The dead and damaged cells leave the skin rough to the touch. Soap addicts will argue there are many products on the market to combat dry skin. Why fix something when it "ain't broke"? Much better to leave it healthy than to try the impossible, revive something that is already destroyed. That is not possible. Give it time and the correct treatment, and the skin may very well surprise you with what it can achieve all by itself *without* help from outside.

The skin can't be treated like an animated object that goes through a process of wear and tear. The skin is a living organ and should be respected and treated as such. It is not an object, and is a lot more valuable. It is an organ with its own renewing or refurbishing mechanism. We can't even try to compete or invent a similar system, as the cells die off continuously and new ones are formed automatically, and this for as long as we live. Soap does not give the new cells a chance to do what they are designed to do, add to the beauty of the skin. They are damaged and destroyed automatically even as they make their appearance.

Like the rest of the incredibly designed human body, the skin is perfect and like the body, quite capable of looking after itself as long as we keep to natural ways of feeding (correct nutrition) and caring for it. Natural delicate watershed dead cells are discarded automatically and new cells are formed continuously that leave the skin soft, supple, and lovely, just begging to be touched.

After not having used soap for some time while bathing or showering, and not using a face cloth, it is pleasant to feel the very different soft velvety texture of your new skin. Believe it or not, another revelation, you don't even want to use a face cloth, perhaps only a soft sponge on a handle for your back. There is no dirt to wash off. What there is to wash of just flows of with the water. If it was essential to use soap, a facecloth, or a brush to wash with, then there are areas on my body which are impossible to reach by hand only, and they must be very dirty after thirty years of not using a brush or a face cloth. The woman or friends in my life have never complained or passed any remark on the state of my personal hygiene, other than welcome positive ones.

We have been so brainwashed by the manufacturers and advertisers of soap products, that the idea of not using soap seems entirely absurd; well perhaps not so absurd. All the chemicals that are expelled through the skin are so delicate and are basically oil-based and therefore water is quite adequate and capable of removing them.

Any engineer will confirm that to remove an oil spill only water is used, and that is all we need to do to our bodies to keep them clean and in a perfectly healthy condition. Use only water.

Soap contains sodas, among other chemicals designed to clean. Skin is very sensitive and it can't tolerate chemicals it is not designed to handle. There are many natural oils and creams available on the market to enhance its natural beauty. In the main, water alone is all that is necessary to look after your potentially natural beautiful skin.

By adding a number of foreign chemicals to what should be just a natural washing with water only process, you are interfering with the ability of the skin to look after itself. After all is said and done, the skin is used to handle anything natural that is thrown at it throughout the ages with consummate ease, without the help of chemicals.

Why not soap? It is commonly known that a woman is as old as her hands and not her face. They don't clean their faces with soap, but with all kind of lotions and potions. Their hands tell an entirely a different story. It is impossible to avoid soap altogether in any normal household. Soap is extremely harsh on the skin, which is simply not designed to be treated in that way. The body as a whole can tolerate foreign chemicals only to a certain extent, and the skin is a lot more sensitive in spite of its amazing ability to withstand the onslaught of the elements. The reason? The elements are natural, chemicals are a different story altogether.

By using cleaning materials we impair the functioning ability of the natural chemicals in the skin as they are completely incompatible, one with the other. Perspiration comes to mind. Could that be one of the reasons why the smell of perspiration is generally so offensive? Surprisingly enough to the uninitiated, it is not the case where soap is off limits. There is no odour.

As stated elsewhere, offensive smelling body odours are the result of a poorly maintained digestive system. A combination of perspiration from such a body and soap residue or antiperspirant causes the offensive odours. The odours from a well-managed digestive system are usually completely benign. This is an experiment that can easily be conducted. A shirt worn by a person who does not use soap and has a clean digestive system can be worn for several days without any odours being detected. This is certainly no fallacy or else I would have noticed that people around me avoid my presence.

Let's perform a little experiment. Have a regular bath and when finished, look back and observed what you left behind. Not a pretty sight, a dark ring above the waterline. I wonder what that could be? Some with embarrassment would say soap. True, but mixed with dirt. Now please explain. If it sticks to the bath, why would the same mix not stick to the skin? Not a pleasant thought. Next step, use a clean light colored or white towel. Dry yourself, where does the dirt go? Only two places, onto the towel and your skin. After two or three days, the towel is in a pretty disgusting state. To clean the bath takes quite an effort and some more cleaning material.

Next step. Follow the same procedure, only this time do not use soap for a few days before you start with the experiment. When finished washing, everything is still sparkling clean. The "dirt" has dissolved in the water as it was designed to do. Should you like, rinse off in clean water and you will be as clean as never before. Now dry off with a clean towel, and use it for as long as you like. There is no dirt to rub off and after three or four days it will still be as clean and spotless as before. How is it possible that a towel can still be clean after three or four days use? Very easy to understand – all you have washed off is natural oil from your skin together with the "dirt," There is no soap residue, the skin is clean, the water is clean, and there is nothing to spoil the towel. Feel free to swap it for a nice fresh one. What about the bath? No more than a rinse will be sufficient, no need for cleaning material. The experiment is over. Guess which of the two experiments will leave you the cleanest, first or second?

It is common for people who do not use soap to look ten years younger, because they love their skin, one of nature's most delicate structures. Soap has a drying out effect on the skin that is easily observable. The designer of the human body knew what He was doing. He provided cleaning material as required, only water no soap.

Nothing wrong with a bit of pampering after a nice leisurely lie in a hot tub. Go ahead, enjoy yourself, and afterward to get clean use warm water only. ***Do not use soap.***

I have another example. I live in a high-rise building. The winds can be testing up there and periodically we have to replace putty on the windows (sealing material) that has come off. I did the job as far as I could reach. The window cleaner, who has a safety harness, happily obliged. Once he had finished, it was cleaning time. Not having given it much thought, I was surprised at the size of the cleaning process. It was major. We ended up scraping the mixture off his hands with the blind side of the knife as much as possible, then used a rag, then hot water and soap. Only then it occurred to me how easy it was to clean my hands compared to the window cleaner who uses soap all day long. I simply wiped my hands clean with a dry cloth. That was it. Because the smell of putty appeals to me, I purposefully didn't wash them. What does that tell you? A naturally kept skin automatically sheds dirt. Nothing sticks to the delicate oil in the skin, not even paint. Handymen will tell you to paint a surface it has to be free of all dirt, oil and must be clean. A piece of sandpaper is needed to roughen the surface for the paint to stick. Don't treat your skin like a surface to be painted.

The manufacturers advertise their soap as the most gentle dirt remover ever, but included are all kinds of lovely smelling lotions and potions. It still remains soap. It is a vast industry and earn huge amounts of revenue. Rather support charity.

I feel compelled to tell the history of my own skin that led to the abolishment of soap anywhere near my immediate environment. More than thirty years ago my skin was rough, dry, and flaky, with some minor spots of what would inevitably have developed into skin cancer, presumably as a result of spending so much time in the hot African sun. To treat the spots I applied some gel made from the Allow plant and they soon disappeared.

Some time later, on the side of my nose, was what at the time I perceived as a serious attack by the enemy – cancer. It was extremely sensitive to the touch, almost as if the skin had already disappeared and I was touching raw flesh. Alarm bells started to ring in my head, some serious consideration and time for some deep thinking had arrived. I decided to put the no soap regime I had been aware of for a long time on trial (without any medical advice, I was convinced their advice would be far too excessive, too much to even contemplate). I stopped washing with soap. It did not take long for the spot on my nose to disappear. Today when my thoughts wonder and I think of that incident, I automatically wonder what the situation would have been like had I continued in the traditional way. I leave that to you to come to a conclusion.

Today, thirty years later, I receive many compliments on the condition of a young and healthy looking skin. Being someone who find creams, lotions, and oils, being rubbed all over me unpleasant, I decided to take the experiment one step further.

I stopped using sunscreen for protection. That was forty years ago, and I never suffered any ill effects, not even where the spots were before, and none since. Once again, it makes sense that the skin has the ability to reconstruct the cells and reconstitute the tissue it needs to renew and heal the damaged areas rapidly, even those damaged by the sun (together with soap). This can only happen once the skin has been allowed to reconstitute itself after having been free of the ravages wreaked upon it by the use of soap, and this may take a while.

Mothers, you have tried it and have seen the results, now start your children off on this important routine at an early age Right from the beginning, after birth, use water only. Pass the benefits on to them and notice the difference.

Under the chapter titled "Toxins" you can read more on how important it is to keep the inside of the body clean of all toxins. It stands to reason that toxins, which are a destructive and powerful enemy, must have the same effect on the skin as it has on the rest of the body. Combine taking care of the inside of the body with looking after your skin as described above. The results can be staggering. *I don't carry any offensive odours with me, else I would have been reminded of such.*

Many decades ago the people from Africa wore the minimum of clothing, certainly no hats, spent most of their time out in the hot African sun and never suffered any sunburn or skin defects. Their beautiful skin was always a talking point. Today their skin problems are as plentiful as any modern city dweller. May I mention that there was no soap available to them, only delicious clean water that could be drunk while they were washing, the same as I have done many times on my many ventures into the natural wonderful outdoors. I believe that by not using soap, the skin can look after itself. *The combination of soap and sun - a deadly one.* Please, I do not want to advocate that anyone follows my example as far as sunscreen protection is concerned, this is my own personal experience as well as others I may have influenced over time.

Many years ago when I still used soap, we were issued with white caps at our hiking club. White does not filter out the

UV rays. All the men with little hair over time developed serious skin problems on top of their heads. Soon after, I stopped using soap and my scalp recovered completely. Years later I met up with one of my old pals. I was quite shocked at the state his scalp was in, raw wounds with bleeding scabs. He was still using soap.

Another plus for the theory of not washing with soap: when we reach an advanced age in our life we develop brown spots on the skin. Leave them to be, they will reach a stage where they can simply be scraped off gently with a fingernail. Should you wash with soap, they will be there to stay and may become problematic. The skin is one of your best friends treat it as such.

Perhaps a suggestion to dermatologists: **Direct some funds towards investigating the theory that it is not the sun that causes skin cancer, but the combination of exposure to the sun, together with the use of soap. NO SOAP PLUS LOTS OF SUN = HEALTHY SKIN.**

I can personally bear the veracity of the following: Where the sun never shines on my body, the skin is distinctly of weaker quality than where the sun shines all the time I am outside. Sun does not kill, it gives life. Why should the skin be any different? The sun has been blamed for something it is not guilty of for far too long.

Chapter 15

HOLISTIC TO THE RESCUE

Hemorrhoids is a subject I would have preferred not to discuss as this is not a medical journal, nor is it a conventional book on health and well-being. The intention was to arouse interest in the reader to become concerned with a more worthwhile improved lifestyle, thus adding enormous value to his/her existence.

But the problem is so prevalent, even if it is completely preventable. It is an alarming fact that fairly young people develop this very unpleasant condition, and the older one gets the more intense is the suffering. The problem will not just disappear, it is there for good unless an effort is made to remove it, but that is the frightening prospect. I have some good news. I can help, so read on, these monsters can be beaten, rather sooner than later. A completely comfortable and pain-free life can still be a reality.

Hemorrhoids are not a subject that is mentioned in polite conversation, but as this is completely private, just between you and me, so here it is.

These dreaded offenders are formed either by a nerve system out of control or enormous pressure applied when constipation is experienced frequently, or by a lifestyle that is abusive towards the digestive system, in other words extremely bad eating habits.

The end of the colon can't perform as is the case under normal conditions. Constant abuse over a long period of time of the digestive system has caused the veins to dilate on account of the enormous pressure that has become necessary to perform a very natural function. It is the pressure on the dilated veins that causes the pain. At this stage, it is not possible to return to a normal condition, they have been damaged beyond recovery.

Unfortunately, there is no cure, treatment or otherwise that can perform that little miracle and don't allow anybody to try and convince you differently. I speak from experience. Surgery is the only way to put an end to this very uncomfortable and painful experience. I endured suffering for many years to avoid *the* worst pain that is possible after surgery. The reason for this incredible pain is that the dead veins, which are at this stage huge, have to be removed surgically, which leaves a very large area denuded of skin, in other words leaving exposed raw flesh behind. The stomach contents are acid laden and when you visit the toilet you can very well imagine what happens when waste touches the raw flesh.

During one of the several times I ended up on the surgeon's table and while still conscious, the wound had to be washed with surgical spirits. That was when I realised why my arm was first strapped to the table, an experience that was a warning of what to expect, hence the reluctance to have the offending culprits removed.

When I finally gathered the courage to challenge the inevitable, some more surprises awaited my unsuspecting mind. During a hiking outing, I mentioned I would not be able to meet a future commitment. People wanted to know the reason. That was when the barrage of sympathy erupted. In my wildest imagination, I could never have known there are so many people who have had to endure this kind of torture. The stories were horrendous, to say the least. One woman related how, while in the hospital bathroom, she heard a woman in the cubicle next door praying that God should mercifully remove her from this ordeal as she could not face another day of this kind of punishment. This torture can carry on for months, a daily visit with Lucifer.

Another told me she had to endure this punishment for three long months – she would bite on anything available and I can imagine a few rolled up towels were destroyed in the process. There were more accounts of suffering, more or less in the same "vein." The reason for the prolonged suffering is that the body automatically heals itself continuously, it is a never-ending process. By the time the dreaded visit to the toilet arrives since the last visit took place, a fair amount of healing had already been completed. Then the acid wash takes place and all the good work is destroyed, well almost all the good work. With a bit of luck a small percentage is saved. The next time around you have some credit in the bank, albeit minute, and every bit of mercy no matter how small is received with gratitude. This can go on for months until the wound is completely covered with a scab to protect the area against the acid. I was due to leave at lunch time to be at the hospital by late afternoon. On my way home I decided I am a coward and would take the easy way out and not report to the hospital. The next few hours were very difficult, and decisions had to be made. In the end, I decided to go through with the procedure, even if it meant three months of sheer torture. I have already had to endure suffering for so many years.

Then my mind did a familiar thing, it started wandering. This is what it does on a regular basis. It surprised me with the unexpected. The word holistic appeared on the radar screen. The authorities at the hospital gave me a mixture to take that evening. While reading the instructions on the label, the word "holistic" (although not mentioned) occurred to me. If at all possible, I do not take anything unless I am convinced it to be as near to natural as possible. That was when I realized the intention was for my digestive system to be cleaned before the operation, understandably so.

Well, if your stomach is empty, number one, you do not have to go to the toilet, number two, why not keep it empty. I am familiar with fasting. I calculated that in a healthy body, where there are no toxins (refer to the chapter on toxins), a wound of that nature would take at the most three days to form a scab. With no food and only water passing through the stomach, the acid (which should be very little seeing there would be no solids to contend with) would be well diluted. If there was no water, so much the better. Most would be lost through urination anyway. So, the chance of nothing passing through, even water, was great. That sounded terrific. Isn't great to be a positive thinker?

The further my thoughts wandered the more promising it seemed, and the whole scenario took on a completely different hue. The scab (at this stage of my life I am an expert on what scabs are all about due to the kind of life I have chosen to live), which is incredibly strong and virtually impenetrable apart from by violent means, should go a long way to protect the wound from being attacked and penetrated by the acid. The prospects looked distinctly a lot rosier than a few hours ago. I was convinced my theory would work. Surgery was nothing new to me, all due to accidents. I was elated and at peace. By this time my stomach had been cleaned and I had a good night's sleep.

Surgery was a huge success. I refused all food and drank only water and lots of it. After two days I was sent home. As was to be expected, the wound was painful, which was mild in comparison to what was anticipated. It was managed with painkillers, of which I reluctantly took as few as possible, and on the fourth day a few fruits were welcome, only as much as needed to stretch the inevitable as far down the line as I possibly could. So far all my theories were just that, theories. Understandably, in spite of my confident state of mind I was still a little apprehensive. What a delightful discovery when crunch time arrived, and there was no pain. At the time I thought that was the greatest triumph of my life; pain is not a welcome visitor under any circumstances and when it is as nasty as this one could have been, it is a reason to feel in a celebratory mood when it did not occur.

Any person who reads this book and has to face this hurdle will have nothing to fear. I strongly advise you take some herbal blood cleanser a number of times, two weeks running before the great event. *This is to avoid infection as much as possible, which is also a source of pain. The healing will be much faster and the scab so much stronger.*

The cleaner the body on the inside, the less chance of infection setting in. Should you have more time at your disposal, use it to better prepare the body by taking the herbal cleanser over a longer period of time. Stretch the fast to four days if you can. After leaving the hospital, ask your pharmacist for a very mild laxative. Under no circumstances must you strain. Look after your best friend at this time (the scab) with great care. *If you want this recipe to work, under no circumstances must you allow anybody to bully you into deviating from this routine. You have your rights.*

I think this message is plain and simple and easy to understand. Within four days the pain from the wound was a thing of the past and I was well on the way to living a normal life that had eluded me for so many years. It is decades later and all is still quite normal.

Chapter 16

INSOMNIA

One will be hard pushed to think of something to compare and enjoy that is more pleasant experience than a good night's sleep, uninterrupted from the moment the eyes close until they open in the morning. Very few folk are lucky enough to be able to claim that good fortune on a regular basis. The rate at which life is lived at present makes that almost impossible.

A holistic attitude towards the problem can be revealing in its ability to bring it as near to normal as one could wish. This will naturally not apply to folk who have suffered trauma of one kind or another, when a more professional approach would be needed to bring the problem under control. Though there is nothing wrong with first attempting to relieve the exasperation the average unfortunate person experiences the holistic way. Holistic remedies are more than merely localized remedies. They treat the body as a whole and are of benefit in other areas of health and well-being as well. Nothing used holistically is ever wasted. Try the suggestions made further on and you may be pleasantly surprised.

The reasons for this malady are myriad, a large number being due to the poor management of one's lifestyle. Far too much coffee, sugary drinks, or drinks containing other stimulants, and out of control stress due to problems that simply do not have an easy solution are also responsible. Here we have a double whammy, and often more coffee than usual is consumed due to the stressful situation. There is much one can do to alleviate the problem by managing the physical side of life, hence providing enough stamina to enhance the level of endurance to handle the situation. This is where a holistic approach to life can play a huge role to regulate and enhance self-control, for instance, diet and exercise.

It goes without saying that for the above to become a reality, the psyche should be at peace as well and if that is not an ideal situation every effort should be made to rectify the malady before an attempt to heal the physical and psychological side.

To go on from there, concentrate on supporting and strengthening the nerves by taking a larger than normal dose of vitamin B which is available in the form of a multivitamin, or a vitamin B complex by itself, obtainable separately from other vitamins over the counter. It is suggested that you take the vitamin B with meals as they are in actual fact nutrition in highly concentrated form. Vitamin B can act as a quick acting remedy to steady fluttering nerves. They are oil-based vitamins and need bile to be broken down, processed, and digested, and thus must be taken after a meal when bile had been released.

Those folk who are living it up a little more than what is considered normal with a hectic social life, whose minds cannot keep pace with this lack of control and who have reached a serious state of confusion, no longer know what is normal. The way back to normality is definitely **not** to take pills to make you fall asleep. These drugs are easily habit-forming and can't solve the problem in any event. Part of the solution is obviously to slow down on your social activities; the other part of the answer is to expand a much higher level of physical energy. This can vary enormously. For the unfit, a fitness program for beginners will more than likely suffice.

The reasonably fit and healthy person, already on an exercise program, can achieve such a level only by an increased amount of sporting activity, far more than he is used to at the moment (these folk seldom suffer this kind of malady). The idea is to exhaust yourself enough to fall into bed at night and sleep. The only problem is that you will probably wake up as soon as you have had a reasonable amount of rest. Your mind has been programmed not to sleep according to what is regarded as a normal length of time, but don't despair.

Remember the mind control system you have mastered by now, apply the principle and start to reprogram your mind in a calculated way. It will be hard work, but well worth the effort in the end. Do not go on to sleeping tablets if you are not on them already. Keep on with the strenuous exercise program, and exhaust yourself every day. Gradually the periods you sleep will get longer and the awake period will get shorter. When you have recovered, the chances of staying on the new exercise regime will be very good. You have actually gained by the adverse experience.

A note of caution - do not get out of bed when you cannot sleep and do more exercises to make you tired again. All that will do is generate more energy, which will keep you awake. Should you already be on sleeping tablets and have not yet relinquished the habit, start the weaning process. Divide one tablet into four quarters and take one-quarter less every few days. Continue until all the tablets have been used up and you will more than likely be free of the habit. For the sake of good health, not to continue with the sleeping tablets is a wise decision, more than likely the most important part of the exercise.

If you are not an active person, now is the time to become active. Start a serious but slow exercise program that suits your level of fitness. Just remember, you must stretch yourself until you are exhausted, no matter how small the effort. You will have benefited both ways in the end. A new fitness regime with all the accompanying benefits of new horizons, seeing your problems in a new light, and realizing there is more to life than just one viewpoint. Apply the same mind-control principle while exercising. Be gentle on yourself don't overdo it, but do stretch yourself. You be the judge, reap the benefits of your efforts. Whatever you do to bring about changes in your body or lifestyle, always try and have fun or at least a lighter outlook on life. Life is meant to be enjoyed.

For those folk who do not really suffer the rigors of insomnia but find it difficult to fall asleep there is some help in the offing as well. Mind control is of some importance. When you find yourself in this situation, it is more than likely that your brain is overactive and it may seem like your mind is in "runaway" mode. This situation could, among others, be due to a poor diet which stimulates your metabolism.

Remember what you have learned from the chapter on the mind. You are in charge, and I am sure you have by now accepted that you and your mind are separate entities and that you are the dominant force in this twosome. Be firm, make your mind understand what is required and enforce the issue. Probably the only time I would advocate an attitude of aggression.

Make sure the room is fairly dark. If you can't find one, cut a mask from any dark soft fabric using several layers if need be. It must be completely dark when you wear it. This can be very important as the mask will play an important psychological role in the process of making you fall asleep. Use the mask only when you can't fall asleep. Eventually when you put the mask on you will immediately feel a sense of cozy comfort and security, a feeling that blocks out interference from the rest of the world. It is important to be in the dark when you put the mask on, otherwise, your eyes will trap some light and hold onto the image. Or put the mask on, open your eyes and then close them again. The subconscious will automatically accept the mask and associate it with sleep, which will help to tilt the balance in favour of falling asleep. It all adds up to building a dominant psychological effect to persuade the mind to fall asleep.

Make sure you are comfortable, not too hot, not too cold. Now is the stage where mind control comes in. **First of all, relax.** Make your mind blank by imagining **your thoughts disappearing into the pillow**. Keep it a blank by staring at the back of your eyelids. All you must see at this stage is black. This is the **most important** part of the exercise. Relax your facial muscles, concentrate on your mouth, your jaw, and in particular the tongue. Check your tongue often, especially in the beginning stages of the exercise. Hold that pose and relax. If you falter don't despair, check what you are not doing right. Just go back time after time until you have mastered the technique. Listen to yourself breathe in a relaxed way, allow your mind to fall in with the pace of your breathing action and simply keep it there. **Do not concentrate,** just listen. The rhythmic atmosphere will have a soothing effect on your nerves, all working together to achieve what you set out to do. It may seem a lot to do and perhaps a little difficult, but it is actually very easy.

Difficulty in falling asleep is often due to a negative frame of mind. Exchange your negative thoughts for more pleasant ones. Think thoughts that make you happy, relish them, bathe your mind in them. Banish the negative thoughts and leave your mind in a happy state.

Nerves that are not quite settled, a condition that is not all that difficult to reach in this day and age on account of poor eating habits, could very well be the culprit that keeps you from having a good night's sleep. If you do not take a multivitamin supplement, now is the time to start taking one with strong vitamin B content. It is important to take it with the *evening* meal. Should you still battle a bit with falling asleep, take the multivitamins half an hour before you go to bed. Important – take the vitamins together with a small snack. Reason: vitamin B is oil-based and need bile to be activated. Bile is only released when food reaches the stomach. Experiment, see what works for you. The vitamin B will definitely have a calming effect on the nerves.

Never underestimate the power of vitamins. Taking vitamins are an excellent way of restoring balances in the body that have been upset one way or the other. Vitamins are not a stimulant, and will not interfere with sleep. With a life that is very demanding, conditions that are not normal for the human system to cope with, not forgetting all the nutrition-depleted foods we ingest, it has become almost compulsory to be on a multivitamin regime with the preponderant ingredient vitamin B, known as food for stressed out nerves. The excess vitamins we take will never be wasted, what is not used in one place will be of benefit somewhere else.

Due to the popularity of coffee, it would not be a waste to stress the important role caffeine plays in the life of a coffee lover who drinks an excessive amount. It could also be a reason why you are not enjoying a comfortable night's sleep. Coffee is a powerful stimulant, albeit one of if not the top-ranking delicacy we can enjoy. It is up to you which of the two you prefer – too much coffee or sleep. It is not often you will be able to enjoy both. I know it is difficult to decide. Caffeine is not a healthy commodity by any stretch of the imagination. I am a coffee lover and being on a health kick, I have discovered decaffeinated coffee is so good these days one can hardly notice the difference. I would also like to stress this does not describe all coffees. There are many different brands and qualities available. I don't think my previous statement will find much favour with the coffee connoisseurs, but try it in any event. Desperate means for desperate situations.

To get back to the, "I can't sleep" issue, enjoy your cup of coffee. Just have it early in the day and make it a special one. Should you have an adverse nerve condition and be able to enjoy a delicious cup of coffee, try the decaffeinated kind. Sugar also has a very powerful stimulating effect so take care not to consume anything containing more than just a small measure of sugar less than three to four hours before bedtime.

All the above exercises will serve a very good purpose in disciplining the mind and eventually your lifestyle. Taking ultimate control of your life that has been hijacked in the name of high productivity and progress, should be a priority which is a God-given right. In spite of all the demands made on us, we still have the right to live a decent and wholesome life.

Make sure you do not eat later than four hours before bedtime. Keep your meals light in the evening, especially protein and carbohydrates. Eat both at lunch time. This could be a little tricky and interfere with your work schedule, but where there is a will there is a way. In our western world with our slightly less concern with discipline, it may sound a little foreign. Perhaps now is an opportunity to fall in line with the rest of the world, for instance, the east, where it is the only way of life they know and definitely the better choice. It is something I have become aware of during my travels around the world.

For optimal health it is generally recommended that one eats five times a day instead of only three; five smaller meals instead of three large ones as is the general custom with nations in the west. In the eastern side of the world, people eat considerably less than in the west. Their food is less stodgy and much lighter in bulk than is the case with the western world. We do not need to eat as much as is the custom in the western hemisphere. A much larger variety of quality foods is essential.

The body needs a huge variety of nutrients, as many as possible, not the bulk we are so used to. With the newly found liberalized thinking process, it will be so much easier to break from the old established traditions as far as eating habits are concerned. Consider having your meal containing heavy ingredients as early as possible, with only a light snack containing fruit and raw vegetables later in the evening.

Drink enough water. A thirst that develops during the night can cause you to wake up. Sensible water drinking is of the utmost importance. Drink a fairly large cup a full two hours before going to bed. Go to the toilet before going to bed, then drink a much smaller quantity of water. A hot drink will also help. Keep some water next to the bed in case you wake up with a thirst, have a drink, and go back to sleep. Try not to think, stay in the sleep mode you are in; if not, try the new recipe again. It will take some effort because nothing worthwhile comes easy. This is a new technique you have to learn and get used to. Above all, remain in a light-hearted mood, no need to stress. Eliminate stress as fast as you possibly can to facilitate healing.

Let's delve a little deeper into the art of sleeping – yes, I think one can very well call it an art, albeit one so many people have a problem with. The serious problem is when victims make the dangerous decision to take sleeping tablets. They are, if not careful, taking on an enemy that will be very difficult to defeat and can lead to devastating consequences. It starts with only one pill and can eventually lead to taking many more per day, a habit that can lead to situations that will make sleeplessness feel like a comfort zone. Sleeping tablets are not a natural commodity. Taking them over a period of time will almost certainly lead to addiction with serious side-effects. The next step is to take some more drugs to combat those side-effects, the beginning of a disastrous lifestyle.

Most people think they are awake much more than really is the case, as the combination of night time, the dark and being half asleep, worries about not being able to sleep, plays tricks on the mind. Relax, even though you are not asleep you are resting, which is just as important as sleeping. Very important, do **not worry** when you are awake. Take charge, use mind control, deny the worrying thoughts access to your mind, replace them with pleasant thoughts to pass through your mind and you will soon be sound asleep.

We do not need as much sleep as we think we do. People need less and less sleep as they get older. At this stage of my life, I sleep between five and six hours per night and I am brim-full of energy. Forget about the old rule that everyone must get eight hours sleep. That one went out the window a long time ago. Children need lots of sleep at a young age; the energy they expend with their tiny bodies far exceeds that of an adult in proportion.

It becomes rather interesting when we take a closer look at the amount of sleep we need to feel on top of the world with energy to spare. It is generally accepted that the brain needs four hours sleep per day to feel completely rested and recharged to perform optimally. Not to forget that the brain is a hard-working organ. It receives instructions from the mind all day long and has to direct them to whatever and wherever they are needed – the mind, mouth for talking, the hands, feet or any other body parts where some action is required, via the nerves.

What happens during this period of rest and recuperation? Like any other part of the body, the brain also suffers wear and tear; the worn cells need to be replaced and general maintenance happens automatically.

Likewise, the nerves which also consist of tissue undergo the same treatment. It is important that the quality of sleep is sufficient and of the highest possible standard to be assured of a clear and well-rested mind and nerve system during the day. Four hours of sound sleep seems to be an adequate amount, with a little extra as a bonus. Who will say no to a little extra sleep? Aim to get yourself into that frame of mind and outlook.

The body is slightly different. It requires at least five to six hours for the maintenance crew to do its work properly. That does not mean that one has to stay in bed for that length of time, as long as the body is restfully occupied. Next time you are awake when you think you should be sleeping, don't worry give the body time to rest while you occupy your mind in some other fashion. The mind is extremely effective after a few hours' sleep, be careful to keep it light on the thinking side. Do something that is repetitive or creative and enjoyable.

Another hint would be to watch T.V. Not too much, and be careful what you watch. As soon as you have reached a state of relaxation, go back to bed without doing any thinking. Put on your mask and go back to sleep. Reading would be another suggestion. Try not to worry (use mind control). Worrying is a powerful, destructive process and will keep you awake. Leave the thinking about your troubles for daytime consumption. There is nothing you can do about solving them in the middle of the night in any event. Enjoy at least that part of your day by spoiling yourself with some well-deserved sleep. Take charge, use the power of your mind to control your thinking and go back to sleep.

In general, we are much too concerned about this matter. Less thinking about sleep, less concern about the lack of sleep, will lead to perhaps less sleep, but more concentrated and deeper sleep. It is far more important to experience deep sleep, albeit shorter and of better quality. REM sleep which translates into Rapid Eye Movement according to the expert.s is vitally important. That is a three-hour plus stint. Some say it is important to experience it during the first half of the night; others maintain the latter half is the recommended time. I used to be a bad sleeper and have found it to be absolutely essential to sleep deep for approximately three hours per night, with one or two extra hours thrown in as a bonus, without it making any difference which half it happens in.

The important point is not to let the concern for sleep become the dominant factor in your life, but rather that you take control and dominate sleep. Once you have tried all these suggestions, it is time to use mind control and enforce it upon your sleeping habits. It may be a good idea to suggest you break up your night into two periods like I have done for many years. I sleep for approximately three hours plus, wake up and do something constructive for several hours, or watch a bit of television when I feel that way inclined, or practice my favourite past-time, positive thinking. This I find really gratifying as my mind is so powerful and fresh after a few hours' sleep the thoughts tend to come fast and furious, perhaps with a bit of fantasy thrown in which tends to happen at night time, but it is up to you to keep your thoughts under control.

I would suggest you refrain from this practice until you are master of your sleeping pattern and in total control. You must be able to say to yourself: *enough, it's time to get back to sleep.* Turn out the light, put on your mask, and wish yourself sweet dreams. Sleep, although absolutely essential for good health, shouldn't be allowed to dominate your life. Worrying about not being able to sleep is a much more damaging factor. You are in charge; sleep can and should be well managed.

Believe it or not, the opposite is also true. Sleeping too much is just another example of a lifestyle which has lost out in reality due to the age old problem, over-indulgence in unhealthy food intake and not enough exercise. Stodgy food not only inhibits the metabolism from operating optimally, but slows it down enormously and obstructs the creation of energy. The body uses the major part of the energy supply to digest food, leaving little for you to enjoy on account of the nature of stodgy food which is completely unnatural, and not at all what the body was designed to handle. Once again we score by eating properly, lose weight, sleep less, and have more time to enjoy the extra and abundant energy.

Does that not sound fantastic? This goes for anybody at any age. While there is still life there is always room for improvement so grab your share of the joy, pleasure, and happiness that is there to be had. **You, take charge of your life.**

Chapter 17

HEARING

Yes, ear candles. Not the usual kind of candle – the solid ones with a wick – but a hollow tube of wax and cloth. The cloth that makes up the wall of the candle is actually the wick. The candle is plus minus two hundred mm long and as thick as the little finger.

This is an ancient natural remedy. It is not quite clear who the first people were to make use of this kind of treatment. It is widely accepted that it originated in the Americas hundreds of years ago. Exactly what materials were used to make the candles is also not known, although it is thought it could have been a dried reed. Whatever it was, it is clear that the principal method of treatment and the reasons for the treatment, is much to our good fortune well preserved.

What are the functions of the candles? The candles enjoy a wide popularity, primarily to remove wax from the ears in a safe and very pleasant way. Apart from that, relief can be had from earache of various descriptions, infections etc., which will become clear later on.

Clever minds have always been around, and to conceive and develop an idea of this kind is nothing short of being brilliant. How the candle works involves a little knowledge of physics, not that the master brain that discovered the process would even have been aware of it. The system operates on the principle of a vacuum, a sealed unit with one opening.

The user lies on his/her side, on a flat surface (the carpet would be a good choice) with a bent arm under the head to act as a headrest. Make sure the bottom ear stays open. The assistant cuts across the center of a paper plate (or any material that will act as protection against falling dust), and inserts the candle through the cross in the plate. An assistant is very necessary as the noise emanating from the burning candle, and heard only by the "patient," is a pleasant crackling sound and it is not uncommon for the person to nod off. Pay careful attention, we are literally playing with fire.

Gently screw the candle into the ear, light it, and make sure **no** smoke emanates from the bottom of the candle. It has to form a vacuum. If smoke does escape, screw the candle in deeper. Proper sealing is essential.

Burn the candle down to about sixty mm from the bottom. ***Do not*** burn the candle any lower down, or the heat may become a little too intense. Remove the stub and douse it in a cup of water that should be kept handy. Unroll the stub and inspect the results.

For children under the age of twelve, only half a candle should be used – the top half, the reason being that the bottom half will get too hot too soon the second time around to have any benefit and this is not ideal. ***Destroy the bottom half.***

The ears have undergone a fair amount of trauma during the process and will possibly not "feel" normal. Occasionally it happens that the inner ear protects itself from the heat and some water accumulates behind the eardrum. It is essential to cool the area behind the ear with a block of ice wrapped in a thin wet cloth, or a small plastic bag filled with water kept in the refrigerator. If not available, make a small bag from the corner of a larger one. Gather the top together with a piece of string or rubber band. This method of clearing the ears of wax is far safer than the more modern method where the ear is syringed, which could be dangerous and should rather make way for the candling method.

To claim that the candles can cure all ailments concerning the ears would be extravagant, but there is nothing stopping a person from trying this very safe and effective method first. The results that were reported over the many years where this method has been in practice are staggering. Some case studies include a mother frantically asked a therapist if it would be safe to use the candles on her little girl's badly infected ear. The infection was so bad, the puss was pouring out of the ear.

The therapist was hesitant to say yes and asked the doctor's advice. The doctor advised that she wait until the next day, hoping the ear would improve overnight. This was late in the day, and mothers being what mothers are, she could no longer tolerate seeing the little girl suffer. After a long discussion, the therapist suggested she use her own discretion. Being an enthusiastic believer in the virtues of the candles, she made the decision to go ahead. Fortunately, all worked out well. The child slept well and the next day she was a whole lot better, with the ear well on the way to recovering.

Another therapist reported she used six candles on a person's ear. The gunge just kept on coming. Inspecting the ear, she could at last see something that was not visible before Using a pair of tweezers, she pulled out a cotton bud that had been in the ear for a considerable length of time. The "patient" did not realize that the cotton bud had separated from the rest of the stem and was left behind in her ear. Moral of the story – do not put anything smaller than your elbow into your ear!

Another more recent case was a keen swimmer, a young lady who sensibly enough used some protection before getting into the water. After getting out she put her finger in her ear and could not feel the plug, assuming the object had come out during the swim. Mother obligingly put in another one. It was only after the young lady realized she was becoming hard of hearing, that candle power was employed. A number of candles were used. What came to the surface one after another were tiny plastic shells, leftovers from the earplugs. They had not been falling out, but had been accumulating in the ears. The drawing power of the candles is immense.

For small children, it is essential to put a drop of soft oil into the ear the night before using the candles (soft oil like almond oil). *Under no circumstances should pure aromatherapy or heavy oil be used inside the ears.* Increase the number of days of oil treatment before candling with the increase of age, up to six days for granddad where the wax has become compacted or hard.

The aged often have severe wax problems and can require several candles to be used, together with lots of patience. Time should not be of the essence and it should not be rushed. At that age, the wax is usually very hard and compacted. The candles can be used once a year, one candle per ear for the average person who does not have any abnormalities, as maintenance. For the less fortunate it can be used as deemed necessary.

Inspect the second candle halfway through the burning process. Should soft wax occur stop the procedure, the eardrum will dry out and start to itch severely, which can be very uncomfortable. Should that happen, a drop or two of soft oil will help to relieve the itching. This could last for several days. A good mixture, but not essential, to relieve the itching would be ten drops each of chamomile and lavender oils per 20 ml of almond oil.

When an object is left behind in the ear, the ear protects itself by allowing the wax to form, hence the wax build up. Another way the ear protects itself is during continuous exposure to excessive noise. The same happens with the frequent use of the telephone. This is noticed when we realize that we can hear better with one ear than the other. One has the habit of using the same ear every time when speaking on the phone.

The way the candling method works is rather interesting. Hot air rises. There is no way for the hot air to escape but through the opening at the top. This rising hot air creates a suction action, which leaves a vacuum behind. This vacuum, in turn, draws air down into the ear which passes through the flame on the way down and the air becomes warm. The warm air vaporizes the wax and is drawn out of the ear. On inspection, the accumulated wax that is visible is not all the wax that was removed from the ear. Some wax turned to vapor is drawn up past the flame and is burned away.

Chapter 18

LOSING WEIGHT

Such an overpowering subject believe it or not is "all in the mind." During the process of getting things right, mind control is of the utmost importance. Make a powerful effort to achieve the best results from that great ally, your mind, which you have by now trained to be your servant. Make sure you understand the relevant chapter. Your mind needs to be convinced that the present status quo is highly undesirable and that the "new you" you envisage is much more in line with what you would like to be and look like, a lot more fun with all the positive aspects to be enjoyed, the only option until your goal has been achieved.

Do not try and lose weight until you have done just that. Then read the chapter on discipline. If you do things in any other way you may lose some weight, and even achieve your goal. It is, however, almost certain you will end up bowing to the very familiar "yo-yo" syndrome and eventually certain defeat.

Your enemy is powerful, of that I do not think you need any reminding. Until you bolster your mind with the power of conviction and determination, I am afraid certain disappointment will stare you in the face. Your weight problem is not your body telling you to overea. Your body has no willpower, neither does it have any say in the decisions you make. It is not your body that has the craving for "food," it is all in the mind. That is where the battle has to be won. Read the chapter on mind dynamics.

To begin with, it is essential to convince your mind that all bad foods containing sugar, white flour, and too much salt, is not for you and should be used sparingly. Too much salt is a certain cause of excess weight.

The ideal way for you would be to use salt as sparingly as possible, and sugar and white flour not at all. They are the greatest enemies of good nutrition, the worst obstacles to good health. Think of them as your enemy number one, whom they certainly are, until you have convinced your mind **they are your worst enemy**, and this should not be mere fantasy, this is for real. *Your mind is very powerful by now and you can rely on it to achieve success.*

At the same time, make friends with the good foods (described earlier) that are available, and apply the same principle (conviction). Become convinced of the merits of what you believe. Make an effort to realize how delicious good food really is. Slowly your mind will accept the new reality, your body will start to enjoy the new natural food designed to feed a natural body. Eventually, you will not believe you were once addicted to food that contained so little nutritional value.

Your mind was for so long bullied and forced into accepting unnatural materials passed off as food when it was really trash. At last, for the first time, your body is being fed properly and you will slowly lose the craving for the foods of inferior quality you forced your body to accept.

Fruit has been documented as a cure for all. Many diseases have been eliminated by using mainly fruit for that purpose. Go slowly on the soft fruits like pears (constipation). People who have been declared terminally ill have recovered completely and lived for many more years after accepting the advice to go onto a main fruit diet, together with enough roughage and acidic fruits to prevent constipation (raw vegetables, whole wheat bread, etc.), together with enough water. It is easy to understand why that should hold so much power.

Looking at it from an overweight problem point of view, the main reason the body has shut down and is completely out of balance is because of an overload of toxins that have destroyed the balance so critically important for optimal metabolic functioning.

The primary function, apart from feeding the body, fruit performs is to remove all toxins from the body. This will take time and it is important to be patient and allow the purifying process to run its full course. Do not try and break records or something ***drastic like colon irrigation, which is certainly not natural.*** It has taken a long time for you to get into the condition you are in, and you cannot reverse the situation overnight. Use the power of your convictions. Fruit is the most balanced of all foods. The diet must also include copious amounts of nuts (almonds being the most suitable) to satisfy the demand for protein. Another excellent suggestion to augment the protein supply is the humble ***whole wheat*** (definitely not white) peanut butter sandwich, should you feel a little peckish. As a matter of fact, at least two slices or more wholewheat bread should be included in your fruit diet to avoid becoming ***constipated.***

A big variety of fruit is necessary, including a good multivitamin, to be sure to cover all the different nutritional requirements to restore the metabolic balance. Not everybody is an expert on nutrition and experts are not always available or they come at a price. Fruit will solve that problem as it is such a versatile commodity and covers such a wide range of nutritional requirements.

Another plus for this diet is the fact that it is so easy, no difficult menus. Nature is accommodating in that respect, and it makes life so easy. There is one fruit that comes to mind I would suggest you leave off your menu at this stage and that is avocado pears. They are extremely rich and may sabotage your efforts to lose weight.

Fruit is not only delicious and refreshing, the variety is enormous. Fruit is naturally sweet and should take care of the natural craving we all have for sweet tasting commodities.

Overindulgence on fruit is not a danger. By all means, eat fruit containing acid like oranges and pineapples. You will soon notice if you are consuming too much acid. (Should it become necessary, a teaspoon tip of celery seeds soaked in a glass of hot water, including the seeds, taken before retiring is a good suggestion). Some oranges and pineapples are extremely sweet with very little acid, and in that case keep on eating.

Another one is bananas, definitely one per day and no more, as bananas are very high in potassium. The heart cannot operate without potassium. One banana per day is absolutely safe and essential. However, the heart also cannot operate with too much potassium and too many bananas can lead to an overload of potassium. In the long run, keep your intake to one or at the most two per day and do not overindulge. Should you feel like more than one by all means enjoy them, even three or four, but then lay off them for a couple of days. A fruit diet is more than likely the easiest way to lose a lot of weight. Overindulgence on the present diet has been the main problem up until now, without the willpower to control your intake of food. Not having to be concerned with eating less gives you one less problem to deal with. You score both ways; eat as much as you like.

Keep to this regime for a week or two then start introducing raw vegetables to your diet. Either include them together with the fruit in a salad, or eat them separately. I cannot think of a more delicious way of eating. Should you feel like eating far more fruit than vegetables, don't hesitate, go for it. As a matter of fact, it is recommended. The easiest way to eat vegetables is via a smoothie as described earlier. Diced vegetables you enjoy together with some fruit juice put through a blender – delicious.

At this stage, you may find you are becoming constipated. A lot of fruit does tend to cause constipation so cut back on your soft fruit intake. Constipation also comes about when a drastic change in the diet takes place, which interferes with the rhythm established when the previous habits were adopted. The whole metabolism needs to change. To mention only one, the endocrine system excreted hormones to cope with the kind of food that was consumed; now that the picture is completely different, the excretions are different. To help the bridging process along, which in some cases can take some time, sometimes weeks, acidic fruit like oranges or pineapples can bring relief. Herbal cleansers (stinging nettle) will also offer relief if taken once a week until things are back to normal. Another suggestion would be to take some natural yogurt, washed down with a little water a few minutes before a meal. Some stewed prunes would also offer a welcome relief. A glass of either pineapple, orange, or grape juice, or a mixture of all three during the evening meal is another suggestion. <u>Remember to drink enough water.</u>

Do not adopt a strict 24-hour time period between visits to the toilet. Strain should be kept to a minimum or it could cause hemorrhoids to form.

Many years ago I attended a seminar concerning health matters. The inevitable subject – constipation – came up for discussion, I was amazed at the response it evoked (proving how prevalent the problem is). The final conclusion was for one to adopt a position as near to a natural one as possible. In other words, the way one would do it in the wilderness where there are no toilets. Bringing to mind the vast experiences I enjoyed in the wilds, it made enormous sense to me. What does one do when back in civilization? Very easy; lean forward as far as possible when on the toilet.

Do not forget to maintain your water intake to prevent constipation and dehydration, as well as helping your body to rid itself of toxins. The changeover has been a bit drastic, and should you start feeling lightheaded, slowly add carbohydrates to your diet: for instance, rice, lentils, four-grain soup, and whole wheat bread, pasta etc. Use equal quantities of rice to water. Cook the rice on a very low heat until just before the kernel bursts, else it becomes mushy. Then add olive oil to taste, only one of many ideas. Find some really nice recipes to help you prepare the whole wheat carbohydrates. If you do not feel lightheaded, continue with the fruit diet.

As a matter of interest, to obtain maximum nutrition, my regular evening meal includes plus minus eight different vegetables, including four different sprouts (in minute quantities raw vegetables contain many times more nutrition compared to cooked vegetables) blended together with fruit juice – delicious. Plus whatever else you feel like. I am not a small man and am brim full of energy. I don't know what it feels like to be tired or below par.

Should you wake up in the middle of the night and become aware of slight hunger pangs, don't rush to the refrigerator and start eating. Drink some water instead. Use your mind power to control those feelings of hunger, denying them any power over you. They are cowards and will soon disappear. *If you have to eat, make it fruit.* It stands to reason that in the past your metabolism has received a certain amount of food, so to reduce weight you have to reduce your food intake. Persevere, your system will soon adapt... and no more hunger pangs.

In the past, your metabolism behaved like a spoiled child, and the slightest craving was satisfied slavishly. Now things are different, a little discipline is brought to bear. When the craving comes, it has to be denied food. The metabolism will get used to the different regime that is in charge and the cravings will soon get the message and subside into oblivion. If you do not have a water filter it will be a good idea to acquire one. Boiling removes chlorine and purifies water adequately, but unfortunately, it does not remove heavy metals. In the beginning it will be tough, but you will be surprised how rapidly your mind will take charge and things will change for the better. Beat this one and it will be a major victory for you. Should you fail, don't stress, keep trying. Treat hunger pangs like any other feeling you have the power to dominate. Once you manage that, you will feel confident you are winning and even welcome the occasional slight feeling of being hungry. Dismiss it with contempt, you are gaining confidence and know you are winning the battle.

Stay away from condiments and other artificial products to make it easier for the body to rid itself of toxins. Here I would like to mention salt. Cut down the consumption as far as possible. It not only makes it more difficult to lose weight, there are myriad undesirable conditions that can be caused in the body by the use of too much salt (as a rule I eat very little salt). Reduce your salt intake to the minimum and discover how delicious food really is. Waterless cooking is a wonderful way to prepare vegetables where no salt is needed.

Remember, you are in charge; be your own person. By now you have learned who and what the most important issues in life are, the ones that serve your best interest. Do not bow to pressure to eat just anything without carefully considering the pros and cons. Peer pressure could very well be a reason (sarcastic remarks). Be proud of what you have achieved. By now it will be so much easier for you to be strong and maintain what you have achieved on account of the powerful convictions you have acquired.

In the beginning, it is common to lose weight at a reasonably fast rate and then suddenly the progress is rather slow, or none at all. Remember, it has all to do with chemicals, a process that is always complicated. The body excretes certain chemicals to handle the kind and amount of food consumed. The drastic change interrupted the process. At this stage, the digestive system has become normal and started exercising control, hence the slower rate of losing weight. It should not be a race against time. You have adopted a natural way of living, the way it should be. After all, your body is a natural creation.

Nothing has the power to provide one with a greater sense of satisfaction than lining up a challenge to conquer, and then demolishing it with relish. Make the challenge interesting; find new recipes; read books new to you on the subject; turn the whole issue into a new project. Allow it to consume you totally. Above all, don't forget to have fun.

Keep the carbohydrates to a separate meal. The next step is to add protein, preferably a vegetable protein such as soya vegetable patties (I have them every day), or soya powder sprinkled over anything you like. Soya is a very versatile product.

Nuts – a hand full of almonds, the best nut for the purpose. Stay on this diet as long as it suits you, and when you have reached your goal and you feel like it, start adding meat to your diet. Stay with chicken and fish, leave the red meat for now as it is a highly toxic commodity.

Once the balance has been restored and the dreadful craving for sugar and salt has been destroyed, it will be much easier to maintain a balanced diet and lifestyle.

Carefully consider what ingredients anything you intend to eat contains, how bad they are, and how much damage they can cause. Use your powerful weapon, mind control.

In the future follow the general trend set out in detail, concentrating on the mental side. Build strong self-esteem, be a winner. Imagine what it will mean to you to know that you have achieved a victory.

Skinny and underweight, that can also be overcome and rectified. Join a gym if at all possible. If not, an exercise bike or swimming is an excellent exercise.

The muscles need to be "woken up" and put to work, together with lots of vegetable protein. You have two choices, soya or weigh (milk). Weigh is very expensive. The use of protein containing steroids is something I would never recommend (unfortunately, very popular), certainly not in the long run. For a short while in extreme cases, yes; certainly not for longer than a month or two just to get the process moving.

VERY IMPORTANT, do not stress as far as exercise is concerned. Read the highlighted section on losing weight and exercise in chapter 21 - SUMMARY. (In short, do not try and lose weight by way of exercising. It puts enormous stress on the heart and could be dangerous).

The secret to success: persevere, do not expect to see any changes too soon, although on the other hand, you may surprise yourself.

Chapter 19

EXERCISE

Although I am not writing about do's and don'ts or about formulae specifically, or different sports in detail, there will be the occasional deviation to be used as an example. There are many publications available on all the different subjects, but here I would make an exception. The intention is to introduce just another easy, free of any expense, and very effective way of keeping the body in perfect condition and somehow completing the scenario, and that is exercise.

The first words that flash through the mind when the word *exercise* is mentioned are pain and suffering, and straining of muscles. It is not only muscles that benefit from exercise, the metabolic rate also benefits. That in itself is a hugely positive note. The organs are wholly dependent upon exercise to perform optimally and to the best of their ability. To rely wholly on the peristaltic movement to keep the organs and intestines in good working order is wishful thinking. Like any other part of the body, the more exercise they receive the stronger they become. Believe it or not, the more they are "shunted" around, the happier they are. Not only do they become stronger, the exercises go a long way towards helping the peristaltic process move the contents of the intestines; at the same time assisting with the digestion, and that is more than just a positive action. They are extremely important to ensure a healthy lifestyle.

One cannot overemphasize the amazing fact that muscles get stronger the more they are put under pressure, even the smallest ones. Consider the eyes. It is difficult to imagine the size of the smallest muscles in the eye. Yet even here it is important to exercise them regularly. We know that staring at a computer screen continuously causes a drastic deterioration of the health of the eyes. It will be difficult for a secretary to do the following: where possible, the eyes can be exercised even while using the computer. Instead of staring at the screen constantly, rather watch the keyboard and move the eyes along as you type. The eyes get an enormous amount of exercise, every muscle, and there are hundreds of them, move with every stroke of the fingers. Each time that happens, the pupils become smaller or larger, and the focal length changes continuously, causing even the eyeball to change size, all in a split second. A muscle cannot wear out, only get stronger with exercise.

ISOMETRICS

No exercise is easier, simpler, and more effective and takes only seconds to perform, with the whole taking no more than a few minutes, than isometric exercises. It is of short duration, but very intense.

This excellent form of exercise, although very old, for some reason is not widely known. I have practiced it on and off over a period of many years and have found it extremely convenient, effective, and time-saving, especially while travelling as you do not need any apparatus. It is completely natural and every muscle and organ in the body can be exercised. It works on a very simple principle. As the word "Isometric" indicates, the muscles work one against another.

Visualize a bodybuilder showing off his physique, flexing every muscle in turn. First one has to learn how to isolate different sets of muscles, and that can be done within seconds. For instance, the solar plexus – bend over slightly, put the hands on the knees, concentrate on flexing the stomach muscles only, pull in the stomach against the spine as much as possible and hold it there for ten to twenty seconds. This is an excellent exercise, not only for the stomach muscles but also the internal organs.

Another is to exercise the arms. Start with the right arm, make a fist while bending the arm and bring the fist up to face level. Grab the right fist with the left hand and try to push the right hand away from the body while the left-hand resists. Not only the arms, but all the chest and muscles across the shoulders and back receive their share of exercise. Hold for twenty seconds.

It is quite easy to work out the different combinations. Visualize a bodybuilder and try and copy what he is doing by simply flexing all the muscles in the body, in turn. This will provide all the muscles and organs in the whole body with a good workout. A bodybuilder has to bring his muscles up to their peak and show them to their best effect and that takes enormous effort. We are not bodybuilders and don't have to go that far. Keep it simple and down to earth, it should be quite enough and don't forget to have fun.

For the really laid back, there is even an easier variation. You do not even need to get out of bed. Upon waking up in the morning, within seconds the whole body can be exercised.

You have just woken up and the first inclination is to stretch. Let this be the beginning of your daily exercises by doing the following, and if you have a sturdy headboard use it as your apparatus. You could also use the steering wheel of your car.

Lie on your back, extend the legs as far as possible, force the toes as far forward and down into the bed as much as you can. At the same time flex the abdominal muscles, not stomach muscles *(the strengthening of these muscles should be of uttermost importance to avoid backache),* the upper leg muscles, then the buttocks, both upper and lower back arching it upwards by flexing all the muscles. Hold for ten to twenty seconds. Relax, then the neck. Pull the head forward towards the chest by clasping the hands behind the head, resist with the neck muscles, and then arch the head backward until it feels the shoulders are lifted off the bed.

While all the muscles in the arms are flexed, push the arms, (which are now next to the body) into the bed as much as possible and arch your back until it feels as if you are lifting off the bed, *flex the lower back muscles until a warm glow is felt.* Next with the arms straight, spread the fingers as far apart as you can and make them curl upwards, at the same time flex the upper arm muscles. Next, make a fist, curl it down and forward, flex the arm muscles, lower and upper, back and front. Flex the stomach muscles again, as often as you like. All the poses must be held for at least twenty seconds. These exercises need to be tried to experience what a great feeling you are left with, and it only takes a few minutes. Everybody can do them. Even the physically challenged will be able to manage some or most of them.

After achieving some success, it becomes a pleasur, and it takes so little time and effort. There are many more combinations. Make life a little more exciting and find them for yourself. These exercises can be done anywhere, sitting, standing or even while walking, or in the motor car waiting for the lights to change. Long distance driving can be a refreshing experience. A word of caution, be discretionary as to which exercises you do while driving. Get into the habit and do those all day long no matter where you are. Nobody need even know what you are up to.

BACKACHE

The "common" backache is a prevalent source of misery everybody who is a victim would like to be rid of. The back muscles are different and should be treated with a little more respect before and after getting out of bed. The back muscles will be stiff from a night sleep; virtually all middle-aged and older persons will wake up with a sore back. The answer is to loosen up before any activity takes place. How? Stretch and stretch and stretch some more.

After a night sleep where our bodies remained in the same position for as long as eight hours causing the back muscles to become stiff, it is important to do the following three steps after the stint in bed.

Step number one.

Sit on the side of the bed. Spread the legs and brace them against the bed. Sit as deep into the bed as possible. Very important: Keep the back straight and sit upright. Stretch the arms sideways at shoulder level and swing vigorously from side to side, feel the blood being forced into the fingers. Try to see what is behind you. Go as fast as you can while all the stomach muscles are relaxed. Repeat as many times as you like, at least twenty times (I do forty times). Do not hold your breath, keep your mouth open, this will force the stale air out of your lungs, and at the same time fill them with fresh new air at every stroke. This is an excellent exercise, not only for the back and lungs but all the internal organs, and extremely effective for folk suffering from constipation. This is an excellent exercise to strengthen the back muscles and re-aligns your spine every day, which is often one of the causes of backache. Don't fuss too much, you will not wear out your spinal cord, but only make it stronger.

Step number two.

Stand next to your bed feet apart, drop the shoulders backward and down, and relax. Pull the buttocks up as far as possible while arching your back. Flex your lower back muscles as tight as possible until a burning sensation is felt. Hold for ten to fifteen seconds, (I do thirty seconds) at least once or as many times as you like.

Step number three.

Try and touch your toes, for most an impossible achievement. It is agony! The first time you may only reach your knees, even the second and third time. At the beginning stages take it easy, as long as you feel some strain at the back of the knees, *it will be enough as long as you make some effort.* By the tenth time you may surprise yourself, and when you have reached the stage where you can touch your toes, it will be so satisfying and for keeps as long as you do them religiously.

Start by standing up straight; make your back hollow by pushing your bottom out while pulling your shoulders back. Flex the lower back muscles until a burning sensation is felt. Hold for ten seconds, put the back of your curled-up wrists on your kidneys, and HOLD THE POSE to avoid straining your back muscles. Now bend over forward as far as possible while pushing the bottom out and only then drop your hands. Go only as far as is comfortable, try and extend the effort every time. It will be painful but only until success is achieved. Then it is a pleasure all the way.

Aim to eventually put your hands flat on the floor (not essential), once successful you can do it for the rest of your life without any difficulty, and the benefits come in generous portions. By doing a little every day you will achieve much in the long run. *To make it easier, bounce the top half of your body up and down, thirty to forty times* and make sure to feel the tendons stretch at the back of the knees.

This is very important to make the back muscles supple so that movement is made easier and relieves the enormous strain the back muscles have to endure. It stretches your tendons from your ankles to the top of the spine. It will always hurt behind your knees. Only dedicated individuals who can touch their knees with their heads will not feel any discomfort, an achievement I once thought I would never enjoy. Now I do it every day.

Another easy way to stretch, or what is also known as lengthening your hamstrings, is to stand about a meter away from a windowsill. Lean forward while with your body is absolutely straight and hold on to the window sill. Lean down onto the sill while your feet remain flat on the floor and feel the pleasant stretched feeling behind your knees. Extend the distance away from the wall until your hamstrings become supple.

Persevere, it's a small price to pay. What can be easier than that all the exercises together took all of five minutes?

I can imagine nine persons out of ten will say before they have even tried, "This is not for me. I have tried it many times and I just cannot do it, it is too painful." Be persistent, surprise yourself. Go slowly, remember – one small effort at a time. You will reach the stage where you will be able to lay your hands flat on the floor. *You need to conquer this monster only once and then it is plain sailing for the rest of your life. Remember that you always get out a whole lot more than the effort you put in.*

The great feeling afterward is worth a king's ransom. That is not too much to ask for a whole lot of wonderful relief from backache. While saying this, *you may still feel some backache after exercise, but as the muscles become supple the pain will start to diminish. Do persevere, don't give up too soon.*

Don't buy into any idea, either self-conceived or from outside, that there is something wrong with your back until you have tried these exercises. Backache is so common it is almost universal.

I still suffer backache every morning after waking up, but within only a few minutes exercising, my back is completely pain-free until the next morning

A common cause of backache is the wrong mattress. Not all can afford an expensive one. There is a reasonably inexpensive substitute – a firm, chip foam also known as a very high-density foam mattress of at least 120 mm thick on a hard base, with a 30 mm soft or low-density foam layer on top. These mattresses need to be turned over once a week.

Unlike our four-legged friends, we walk upright with all the body parts hanging from the front, with the spine holding it all together. To enjoy a comfortable existence, it is important to keep the core muscles *(all the muscles around the midriff, front, sides, and back)* in good condition. The most important are the **abdominal** (not stomach) muscles between the hip bones. Strengthen them by flexing them several times a day as severely as you can whatever position you may hold at the time/ Nobody will even know what you are doing. This exercise, when successfully practiced, will help enormously to rid your back of any pain.

While relaxing, always sit Full Square on a chair, never on the side or on one buttock. The spine is of very complex construction and should be treated with the necessary respect and consideration. The above may sound like a huge amount of advice, but when practiced it will soon seem more realistic and well worth the effort to beat this awful problem.

Using the mind power technique, learn to flex the abdominal muscles at all times. It will not take long to achieve success, eventually you will automatically exercise muscle control without being aware of it.

Many people suffer painful backache occasionally on account of the vertebrae that "slips," for want of a better word; or the back is "out" as it is commonly known, and only the victim will know how painful that can be. To line them up again is relatively easy.

Lie on your side with the bottom leg straight, the top one pulled up at a right angle. Have a friend kneel in front of you, with his knee pushing on top of your angled one, holding both hands one on top of the other against your shoulder. With one almighty shove, push the shoulder against the floor while holding the knee firmly on the floor. This must be done with a snap action. Repeat the exercise on the other side. The pain should be gone instantly.

I have devised a method to attain the same results on my own. There is a heavy cupboard at the bottom end of my bed, (a heavy wooden queen size one), with a small passage in between the two. I lie on my side, wedge the top knee under the bed, which is just the correct height, twist over backward, take hold of the bottom of the cupboard and perform the required snap action, with perfect results. Repeat the exercise by turning around and do the same for the other side. *Please remember you perform all these exercises at your own discretion.* (I have not had reason to do this for a very long time, ever since I have been doing the exercises described above).

If you do not suffer from backache, do the swing exercise anyway. You will feel great and avoid suffering backache in the future. Muscles are begging to be stretched, that is what makes such a superior exercise regime so important, and all this in a matter of two to three minutes. *Life can really be tough at times.*

I personally do not follow a strenuous exercise regime as I no longer participate in any competitive sporting activity. I do these exercises before and after getting out of bed in the morning, and go to the gym three times per week for a light workout. It is important to give the cardiac exercises preference. That I do on an exercise bike for twenty minutes, and various exercises on the machines. Walking is still a passion with me and I walk as often as opportunity allows. My body has received so much exercise all my life long, it is still in very good shape. All it needs at this stage is a mere maintenance program.

Should you never have indulged in any exercise program before and you are a member of the older generation, take it slowly. You will have to trust your own judgment on this one, and perhaps the opinion of your personal physician would be advisable.

A word of caution. Should you be one of the unfortunate victims with a serious back problem who has perhaps undergone surgery, rather seek expert advice as to what extent you can perform exercises with relative safety that will be of benefit to your back. These are mere guidelines and you will have to assume full responsibility when you decide to perform any exercises. Anybody can do some exercise, no matter what condition their body is in.

Stretching together with a little stamina exercise, for instance, walking or an exercise bike, combined with healthy eating habits, are quite adequate for optimum health, provided you are not overweight. If you are overweight, you need to slim down first to achieve some benefit. *Allow me to reiterate, once again, the fact that diet is the most important of the two. Slim down first, then exercise.* Nevertheless try the exercises you can manage anyway, as some are better than none.

Feeling tired after coming home from work, no energy, having supper in front of the TV before going to bed only to be still tired waking up the next morning? This can be changed overnight.

To bring about a change, oxygen is needed to be converted to energy, and to achieve that it is necessary to move. When the body moves, muscles are activated. Oxygen is the essential fuel that makes the energy to move the muscles Let's see how it works.

To start with, a short walk around the block, nothing strenuous, leave that for later, is all that is needed. The moment the muscles are operating, the heart rate increases, and the blood rushes through the body. At the same time, another action comes into play. The lungs work faster. It sucks in oxygen, which is processed and passed onto the blood in the form of energy, which is moved to every muscle in the body, including the brain. Automatically you feel energized and much refreshed.

Both instances have a compacting effect. Continuing with the first situation, you feel a little worse every day. The eventual outcome is a visit to your doctor for a tonic, an artificial remedy which will offer only temporary relief and not change the situation to what should be desired.

With the new regime, the impact is equally intensive to the previous situation, but only in a positive way. Remember to breathe deeply all the time while walking – *more breathing more oxygen more energy.*

A small improvement every day will eventually lead to huge gain. The more you do, the more you will enjoy the benefit of the exercise. One step at a time, you will experience a complete turnaround as to how you feel.

Allow me to mention a very important malady that strikes mainly old people and women in the particular: Osteoporosis – the lack of bone density a condition that is becoming far too prevalent.

It will leave you debilitated and a simple slip and fall can break several bones and even cause death. The main cause of this disease is inactivity as well as poor nutrition. Vitamin D plus Calcium and magnesium can play a role in preventing the conditions, *but vigorous exercises remain the main preventive measure. The harder the body works the stronger it becomes.*

Chapter 20

RETIREMENT

Retirement is a period in life most of us look forward to with so much anticipation. For some, the dream comes true, but unfortunately for most it stays only a dream. The reason: lack of planning or no planning at all. After working hard all your adult life you deserve to have some time you can spend doing what you always wanted to do.

Your planning should start at an early age and take into account the fact that inflation is one of the biggest enemies of our time. So it is imperative you consult with a financial adviser as soon as possible, the younger the better. Unfortunately, young people usually view such advice as superfluous. It takes time and experience to understand how fast time passes by; the days are eaten up as though there is no tomorrow.

Eventually, the benefit you could have had for the same amount of money is so much less. What could have cost perhaps a small amount per month while still young, will cost many times more as you get older for the same benefit in the end. Not to make provision for such eventualities makes bad financial sense and poor judgment on the part of anyone who is serious about his or her future. Do not fall into the trap of thinking "tomorrow is another day," or because you are still young there is plenty of time left to think about things that will matter so far into the future. Young people take note – time can be your friend or your enemy, the choice is yours.

So often you hear the expression "age is only a number" when old age becomes a subject for discussion. On the other hand, any age is a number for that matter. Or "you are as young as you feel." The one that appeals to me the most is to ***"always feel young and full of energy." That is very possible, (ask me I know)*** but you have to prepare for such a luxury. To expect to simply receive such good fortune without effort is, unfortunately, not possible. Even if you are financially secure, your physical condition also plays a part. Like all good things in life, you have to do some work and make some sacrifices to achieve any objective, and this one is no exception. Making sacrifices can be great fun. The mind and body are so constructed that any effort completed satisfactorily is beneficial and always ends on a positive note; and what can be more pleasing than success, not only financially but physically as well? A good balance of mind, body, and soul is essential at any stage of life, and no less so to be able to enjoy well-deserved happiness during old age. The chapter on nutrition and toxins will go a long way towards helping you understand how the body functions in a very easy and simple way.

On an even more serious note, albeit not a pleasant one that will affect all of us, is the expression "old age is not for sissies." The better one's defenses are prepared for this onslaught of nature, the better one will be able to handle this period more comfortably. It can be a substantial length of time and a large part of one's life. It is not necessary to end life in the poor house, in a tiny room in some backyard, or in a crowded home for the aged where old folk sit with blank stares waiting for the inevitable. What a sad scenario. Be prepared for when the time comes. It waits for no one and is on nobody's side, but there is enough time to prepare provided you make good use of the time you have available. It is not uncommon for people to live for fifteen or more years during the period known as "old age." When you are properly prepared, this can be a very rewarding and enjoyable time of life.

On the other hand, should you be ill-prepared, the same length of time can be an interminably long period of misery and unhappiness when you will wish the end would come sooner rather than later. To be of ill-health and unable to afford what your heart desires, or even the basic necessities of life, make the days feel like they will never end.

Preparing the mental and physical side of life to be able to cope with old age is equally important. Here the body and mind work in tandem.

A sound mind is much more comfortable in a sound body, and consequently is much more successful at maintaining a healthy attitude which is more important during this time of life than any other. Life can be a whole lot of fun during old age, often more than you ever dreamed possible. Recently there was a report on local television of a ninety-two-year-old gentleman who completed a one-hundred-and-ten-kilometre cycle race, and not an easy one at that. He did not win but finished, and that is most important. What is so remarkable was that it was the eighth time he has achieved this incredible feat.

Yes, life can be great at any age. The secret – never give up on any activity you practiced with great enthusiasm during your lifetime when you get on in years. It can be as much fun towards the end of life as when you were young. Take care not to think: *well I have done it for so long I deserve to have a break.* This can be a highly-flawed decision. The body tissue is not as resilient as it used to be, a period of inactivity at that age will cause the texture to deteriorate very quickly, and to retrieve what you had before may not be possible. Such a decision can be regrettable. Why take a break from something you enjoy so much? Be warned, the break often tends to become permanent. The body and the power of discipline are not as strong as they used to be, and to start again can be very difficult. To continue and not take a break is the sensible thing to do.

It is encouraging to encounter older people who still live life to the full. At the gymnasium where I have a lot of fun there are, I am tempted to say, several "old gentleman" but forget the "old," at eighty-plus they are an inspiration to all of us. To see them still have a workout is phenomenal. Not all are as motivated as these gentlemen, but it is essential that the body is kept active.

When muscles and tissue are not exercised regularly, or at least kept active on a regular basis, they are not very happy and will show it pretty soon. We will start feeling the difference. When you exercise regularly the benefits are enormous. Do not forget nutrition. Good nutrition will automatically help to preserve and keep the tissue young. Life can be so incredibly beautiful at any age, more so at an old age when we take the opportunity to make the difference.

When I observe older people, and I see a lot of them during my daily activities, one can almost see and feel the regret from the ones who did not care much about looking after

themselves, almost as though they have given up hope of anything exciting ever to come their way again. That need not necessarily be the case.

Recently I met up with a gentleman I have seen before in a restaurant but have not spoken with. This happened in a shopping center and it was clear that he felt the urge to speak to someone. I love old people and was glad to oblige by allowing him to talk. What he had to say would not make for worthwhile reading, except something he repeated a few times and that was: "every night I go to bed I hope I will not wake up in the morning."

What was discussed in the previous paragraph explains it all. Considering his stature, size, and weight, if it were not for the obvious way his health was neglected he could have been in a much better state of health and a much happier person (imagine the difference). When I saw him in the restaurant the time before, I noticed what he was eating (which happens all the time due to my interest in the subject). His health was generally sadly neglected. To think something as basic as poor nutrition was responsible for the sad condition his life was in. Thinking about him later I became convinced it would have been possible to turn his condition around for the better with proper nutrition without much effort. I would have been eternally grateful for the opportunity to take care of a situation such as that.

The mind can be kept alert and active to a ripe old age. Keeping the brain cells active and on the go continuously will add extra fun to life when we get older. Every challenge successfully completed means so much more to a positive atmosphere. There is nothing a wide-awake mind enjoys more than to be challenged, more so at an advanced age. It is incredibly gratifying to see an older person enjoying life, full of fun, mind alert, quick on the uptake. It is not reserved for the privileged few only; most people can enjoy such a state of satisfaction.

I have known some folk who told me their minds are sharper and more alert than when they were employed. During their working career, they were not required to stretch their thinking ability. Subsequently, they became involved in activities that required them to do just that with remarkable results, and they are elated with this new

discovery and how much pleasure they derive from life now that they are retired.

I repeat – preparation for this time of life must **preferably** begin at a much younger age. Young is, of course, relative, and so will be your success, it depends on what your understanding of being young is. One can start at any age. Any activity that challenges the mind and body to achieve a reasonable level of fitness in both respects does not mean you have to achieve athletic status or become a super brain. Anything positive is welcome. Combine that with healthy eating habits and life can be a wonderful experience at any age.

This should be a happy and joyful time of your life, not to be looked at as a period of idly passing the time; the human body is not designed for that purpose and the results will soon show. As mentioned earlier, it is designed to work. Remember the human body gets and stays strong only by being active, and that includes exercise.

Don't forget some light-weight resistance exercises. How much weight, how much exercise? That depends on age and at what level you desire to be active. It is entirely up to the person involved, with a gradual increase in intensity.

As mentioned before, one should bear in mind it takes more effort to regain some of the fitness lost due to an interruption of the exercise regime as one gets on in years. Try to keep to a regular exercise program without interruption, which by this time should not be difficult to maintain; nothing strenuous if you do not so desire. Strenuous exercises are not essential to stay fit and healthy. Just remember, do not try and fool yourself that your diet is far more important. Don't overlook walking as an exercise with a little lightweight training thrown in. When doing exercise with light weights, it is reasonably safe to simply do any movement you feel like doing; just go slowly, warm up a little and use your imagination. The size of the weight is very important. Do not push too hard, rather too small than too big, depending on age and the level of fitness from half a Kg upwards. This advice is meant for the relatively inactive folk. The fitness gurus will know what they prefer and what is safe for them to handle.

We never forget to breathe, but what we do forget though is to do some deep breathing. It is essential the stale air in the bottom of the lungs is expelled. Air does not only become stale, it is alive and like anything that is alive, when it dies, it putrefies. Deep breathing should ideally happen several times a day, more so when exercising. Use the diaphragm when you inhale, draw the air in as deep as possible with the help of the stomach by pushing it out, hold it for a few seconds then breathe out. Do this slowly, or else one might become lightheaded. Refer to the chapter on oxygen to learn more about the importance of breathing properly.

There is no reason why we should lose our mental mobility when old age makes its presence felt; our mind can remain sharp as we get older. Recently I had reason to visit an old age home, better known as a residence for senior citizens. I think I prefer the latter. What perturbed me though was what I saw as I walked inside. There were a large number of elderly folk sitting against the wall around the room staring into space, doing absolutely nothing. I could only put it down to poor efforts on the part of the management of the establishment. Outside there was a beautiful bowling green, large gardens, all very pleasing to the eye – except all were deserted. Should one have the desire to reap some benefit for mind, body and soul, the opportunity was there. Everything was in place to make old age interesting and full of fun during the last few years left.

What I understood was that the local clinic was a very busy place. Too much idle time to pass and no exercise, both mentally and physically, a lethal combination. When we reach those years, it is imperative we keep our body active and faculties occupied. Our resistance wears out much faster and we lose strength rapidly should we do nothing. On the other hand, keeping active with the purpose of staying young for our age is not difficult. Nothing earth shattering is necessary and whatever we do, that will commensurate with our age. Perhaps the management is too busy to make the necessary difference. Here is an opportunity for a person who has the necessary experience and organizing ability to make a difference, by taking a hand in making the world a better place for his fellow residents.

The brain is not a muscle, but it reacts in the same way. The more we exercise it, the stronger and more flexible it becomes. It is not important what we do, as long as we put the mind under pressure and stress, with thinking that is, not worries. There are many different activities available, many books written on the subject, as long as we have to think. Work the brain, it gets tired just like the body; have a break, a rest, but do persevere.

It is strange how the mind works. At first a challenge is difficult, then it becomes easier, then we get used to it, then we start loving what we do. Eventually, the very thing we were so reluctant to do takes hold of us and we cannot get enough. It only takes a small step to make a start. It is well worth the effort. Do not be surprised when you discover that your mental ability and memory improves to an unbelievable degree.

Allow me to mention what I do to keep my mind sharp. I have always enjoyed a love for mental arithmetic. To begin with, I suggest the following: Make a long list of two sets of numbers, multiply them with a calculator and write the totals down and forget about the calculator. In the beginning, keep to the lower numbers, i.e. 15x17 = 255. Break the numbers down and multiply them mentally, i.e. 10x17=170 + half of 170 = 85, 170+85 = 255. Increase the margin of difficulty continuously. Another example: 32x46=1472. 32x100=3200 divided by2=1600 – 32 four times, or 4x30 = 120+8 = 1472. Always find the core number: 100, 50, 20 10 etc. and work from there. This is one of my favourite pass times.

I am acquainted with two people of around eighty years of age. Every time I see them it occurs to me how agile their minds are. Their secret? Crossword puzzles. Neither has any education worth mentioning, but their general knowledge is remarkable with no perceptible slowing down as they got older, always alert and ready with a worthwhile answer. Refer back to the chapter on the mind to read more on this subject. Yes, your quality of life need not suffer the same fate as the years of your life. Be careful when you make the choice where to spend the last years of your life. They could be the best and most interesting years, or long and boring.

This is a time in life that holds a tremendous amount of fear for many, if not for most elderly people. Here I specifically want to refer to the fear of loneliness. For example, losing a beloved spouse. The magnitude of the adjustment is not understood by anybody who has not been through a similar experience. Should you have studied the material thus far and are persuaded that it has merit, I am convinced you will feel considerably more confident facing the future. Younger folk, if you follow the recipe you should have no fear at entering what could be a very difficult or the most enjoyable period of your life.

For our older friends who are already there or are approaching that stage in life, loneliness can be a daunting prospect to face. Here I refer mainly to the women folk. Men must realize that life primarily favours the male side of society, while women are much more vulnerable. Where men can live quite happily on their own and do not need company on a constant basis, women are different. Because they are more vulnerable, sympathy and a word of encouragement are usually warmly welcomed.

Following the preceding suggestions should go long way towards allaying their fears by forming a more positive mindset and building confidence that will take them towards a more independent attitude. Following the trend generally suggested so far should go a long way towards achieving just that.

When considering remarriage to alleviate loneliness, a bold move that needs careful consideration, the difference in personalities not taken seriously, or not even noticed in the rush to acquire a new partner and the prospect of a new relationship, can lead to a sticky situation. Life does not get easier as we get older, and requires a lot of wisdom and careful negotiating of obstacles to ensure a fair amount of happiness. At this stage of our lives, we are so entrenched in or own quirks, habits, and customs we have acquired or accumulated over the years. These, together from the other side, can make a new relationship a strained affair and not the happy a one we so looked forward to. It can sometimes be very difficult, if not impossible, to adapt to new rules and regulations. When we make the effort to be accommodating, it will be under a certain amount of duress and lead to an even more stressful situation. That can make life very unpleasant, sometimes completely unbearable. For most of us to force ourselves into another drastic change at that time can simply not be an option. The only way out is to just grin and bear it, with two very unhappy people, not the desired way of life we anticipated.

The alternative: do what women are very good at and form "alliances." Move in together, create enjoyable activities you can practice together, travel together, and so on. It is not necessary to suggest a list of such activities, there are so many to choose from. Having worked through this material it should not be difficult to find them, using your new enlightened and very much more capable faculties.

Chapter 21

Highlights

SOME POINTS TO PONDER

To overcome a severely addictive habit such as smoking, *together with the mind control* process you have by now adopted, add the weaning system. Be patient and try and achieve your goal over a long period of time. Calculate how many cigarettes you smoke per day, eliminate only one per week. Be patient, don't rush the process; you may have indulged for a very long time.

The same goes for any tablets or drugs you know are harmful and you would like to stop using. Your body will be none the wiser when you deprive it very slowly of the substance you depend on to survive.

HELP FOR THE ELDERLY

I have often come across elderly persons (elderly can range from any age, sixty and older) who obviously are not in a comfortable situation health-wise. They are not sick or ailing from any malady in particular. Physically, they are simply not in a happy place at that moment in time.

Their skin colour is perhaps darker than what should be for their particular skin tone. The skin is rough, sometimes to the extent that lesions are visible. Their eyes are duller than they should be. It is obvious to a trained eye that the kidneys and liver are finding the going rather tough, and need some assistance.

If this is a relative or someone you are fond of, give them something they will remember you by.

Guide them along a suitable line of conversation (it has to be done very diplomatically), and when the opportunity arrives I suggest the following.

Take some Vitamin C 300 mg. (milligram) to strengthen the arteries and heart muscles, and Vitamin E 300 i.u. (international units) to clear the arteries of cholesterol. This will make the heart's job to pump blood through the veins so much easier.

Take some herbal blood cleanser, twice per week for two to three weeks. At the same time, go onto a pure fruit diet or as much fruit as possible for a week. After that, should it be convenient, cook all their vegetables the waterless way. It would be preferable to eat most of their vegetables raw, together with enough fruit. Two slices of whole wheat bread to keep the digestive system functioning and **prevent constipation.** For the time being, stop eating red meat altogether, not forgetting a mild exercise program like walking.

Do not use soap at all, and should there be any lesions on the skin present, simply leave them be. By not using soap, they should disappear soon enough (read the chapter on skin and soap).

The whole idea behind this treatment is to clear the vascular system of all toxins and make it easier for the liver and kidneys to function. The turnaround time will be astonishingly short. *Give them more than merely a gift; give them a new lease on life. Surprise them and show them life can be somewhat better, even at their age.*

Imagine what it will mean to you knowing that you were responsible for the improvement to their lives.

LACKING ENERGY

The ever-present feeling of being run down, listless, lacking enthusiasm for anything that requires physical movement: if that describes how you feel, then there is nothing "wrong" physically, but a whole lot metabolically speaking.

The vascular system is so clogged up with toxins it is not possible for the blood to supply the necessary nutrition to the cells and tissue in order to create the energy the body needs to operate.

This can easily be put right, and a quick fix is possible. As in the case of the elderly mentioned above, apply the same treatment: first the blood cleanser, then lots of fruit for a week; but don't stop there, continue with more fruit in the diet as a matter of course. A generally more improved diet would be recommended, not forgetting to do some walking on a regular basis. Keep an eye out for the signs of constipation due to the intake of a lot of fruit, and if necessary vend your way to some herbal remedies.

AIR CONDITIONING

Air conditioning puts the metabolism under severe stress. When temperatures are high and for several reasons we make life very difficult for ourselves, we dash for the first available airconditioned building. The metabolism is a finely tuned machine and having adapted to the hot conditions outside, suddenly without warning it is subjected to enormous change in temperature. What are you doing to your precious body? Not even this miraculous, finely tuned machine, can cope with such a drastic change and punishment.

More often than not, no sooner has the metabolism adapted to change when the whole process is thrown into reverse. The effect it has on the body is dramatic, to say the least. An enormous amount of energy is consumed in the process and before long fatigue sets in. Every single part of the body is affected by this drastic extreme back and forth changes. Observe those folk who are spending so much time and energy dodging the heat. There is certainly no sign of joy; rather one of frustration and eventual exhaustion.

It would make a lot more sense to learn how to manage the heat and enjoy the warm summer days. Psychologically, we are automatically averse to hot weather, avoid the outdoors and so deprive ourselves of a lot of pleasure that could have been enjoyed by learning how to manage high temperatures. Don't forget, it is all in the mind. That is where the major part of the change has to take place. Remember mind control. Unfortunately, it will take more than just saying a magic word to make it all happen in an instant; it does require effort.

We can, by cooperating with nature, make life a lot more comfortable during the hot summer days. First, we should dress sensibly, wearing only natural fibers such as wool or cotton. These natural fibers, which are not influenced by temperature, absorb the perspiration, and because it breathes, the moisture passes through to the outside where it evaporates when it comes into contact with the air creating, a cooling effect and leaving the body a lot cooler.

Synthetic fibers are vitreous by nature and have a metallic quality that does not breathe or absorb moisture, instead, it traps the warm air and the unabsorbed moisture causing the body temperature to increase unlike natural fibers that do absorb moisture and stay cool. It envelops the body and not only keeps the body hot, acting like an oven, it actually generates more heat which is higher than the ambient temperature and far higher than the body temperature, creating conditions that under extreme circumstances can be dangerous.

Just follow the wise old lady nature, she thought of all eventualities and provided solutions for our problems. Forget about air-conditioning, get used to the natural heat and atmosphere. Another unsound idea to stay cool while walking in the sun is to strip off clothing. The direct sunlight is extremely harsh and heats the body up, and eventually fatigue sets in. Keep the body covered on hot days unless you are sunbathing.

This is particularly evident when walking trails. A good leader would always make sure all his charges are suitably dressed to keep potential problems to a minimum during the hot summer days. Overheating or heat stroke can be serious, especially in arid areas where water is sometimes at a premium, the only commodity that can prevent a potential disaster from becoming a reality.

Keep to light-coloured clothes that reflect heat, unlike darker colours that attract and absorb heat. I have witnessed this phenomenon many times where novice hikers, perhaps out of ignorance, did not obey this particular rule and had to pay the price, fortunately never fatal, but always serious. This usually happened only once to the same person and those who witnessed it. I enjoy my outdoor activities in warm weather conditions and have never had a problem, and I really enjoy being out in the hot African sun covered completely in cotton garb, except for my arms which are always bare.

What a difference the correct choice of clothing can make. Cooperate with nature and you have the world at your feet; many years of enjoyment, compared to being too careful to venture outside, missing out on enjoying nature. Life is designed to have fun, make the most of it while you can.

A common fault practiced widely, is to drink ice cold drinks or take a cold shower during hot spells. You are actually declaring war on yourself. The first thing the doctor does when things are not well with the body is to test the "core temperature."

Should you apply or practice these extreme cold remedies to hot situations inside and outside the body, you are forcing the core temperature off balance. The body immediately responds by generating more heat to restore the balance. Perspiring profusely after taking a cold shower on hot days is another example of nature's reaction to disturbing the balance Remedy? Take a warm shower on hot days.

The exact opposite happens when you take a warm shower (instead of a cool one) or take warm drinks. The body applies the same principle. It cools the body down to restore the core temperature, which controls the body temperature, hence the feeling of being cool. I practice it all the time and enjoy enormous comfort during hot weather.

Another very common mistake repeated ad nausea is to drink ice water during hot spells. <u>"I keep on drinking water but I remain thirsty, how is that possible?"</u> Very simple: The same principle mentioned about a shower above applies in this instance as well. When you pour the ice cold water down your throat, the overheated tissues clam up. It can't absorb the liquid; the liquid simply passes through and you urinate a lot more than usual. Drink the water at ambient temperature and your thirst will soon be a thing of the past.

DEHYDRATION

You have been to the gym, forgot to drink water, or not enough. You try and compensate. After going to bed you soon wake up thirsty and drink some more water. Not long, and you are awake again; the performance repeats itself over and over and you have a bad night.

The body needs an adequate supply of water to function, more so when it is under stress. When the supply runs out it starts to draw from the reserves that belong to the tissue, leaving the tissue in short supply. The nerve endings in the dry tissue become "irritable" and cause you to wake up.

The tissue takes many hours to absorb enough water to become hydrated again. It is important to drink enough water **before and during exercise;** at the same time do not drink too much.

Dehydration can have serious consequences and should not be taken lightly, particularly when the level of activity is high on hot summer days. Equally so is over-hydration, when too much liquid is taken. It is advisable to seek advice from a sport body that is concerned with the particular sport you are involved with, especially sport played at a high level of activity, like running and tennis. My advice is to drink small quantities regularly.

Drinks that will replace the electrolytes lost during practice and play should be investigated as well. This is a very valid point. The body uses nutrition continuously, more so when performing strenuous exercises. Proper formulated drinks are available for sport enthusiasts. To remain on the natural track, the most nutritious and still the most wonderful natural food available to man is good old honey diluted with water, my ultimate favourite.

For energy expenditure on an average everyday basis, nothing more than a healthy nutrition enriched lifestyle is necessary; in other words, ordinary healthy food. Stodgy food is of absolutely no benefit to anybody, especially during hot spells. The metabolism has a mountain to climb digesting it under ideal conditions, imagine how it suffers trying to cope under extreme conditions.

VITAMINS

As mentioned before, one is inclined to consider one vitamin or a particular nutrient above another. They are all vitally important for the metabolism to function and perform optimally, for instance, potassium. Your heart will function perfectly normally when the potassium is running low until it is depleted altogether, then fibrillation will set in, and the heart will start racing out of control with consequences that can be catastrophic. Make sure you get your necessary dose of potassium by eating at least one banana per day. That will supply you with all the potassium your body requires.

Most organs need one individual main vitamin, with several others in smaller values with their own individual combinations. Several organs may need **almost** the same combination of vitamins, but with different values.

Vitamins are on the whole, within reason, harmless provided good sense prevails and the individual does not see vitamins as a means of experimenting to improve his/her health and become reckless in the process. Always seek expert advice; it will prove to be not only more profitable but you will find success much sooner in the process. It would be no more dangerous than overeating. You would simply be producing expensive urine.

When you feel all is not well health-wise, and it is not yet time to approach a physician for advice, try the natural route first and pay the local health food store a visit. Like everything in life, health stores are not all up to standard, but hopefully you have by now done the rounds and found one that you feel comfortable with to ask for advice. Be careful you are not spending more money than you need to, leaving with a lot of unnecessary items. Read the instructions printed on the container carefully.

The health industry has advanced tremendously over the past decade and has kept on par with the development of allopathic medicines.

A number of ailments of a mild nature can assail you. An imbalance may occur in the body and a simple course of multivitamins could do the job of correcting the imbalance.

Another excellent product line is a whole range of tissue salts available that can be very effective. Selecting what you need is as easy as reading on the container what the particular remedy is meant to cure, and is inexpensive. The range consists of twelve different bottles, each of which covers three or four different ailments. To mention just one as an example: you may feel a bit lethargic with no energy, or slightly lightheaded, symptoms which are usually associated with a light case of anemia, lack of iron in the blood. That does not necessarily mean that you have a lack of iron in your system, it simply means that your blood does not absorb all the iron available. This is where tissue salts come into the picture, which acts as a catalyst, number 2 container in this instance.

Place one tablet under your tongue a few minutes before each meal. There is a membrane underneath the tongue where the remedies are absorbed directly into the bloodstream, hence the speedy reaction.

These remedies are made of natural ingredients, are non-toxic, and completely safe to use. It is not possible to overdose. Should you feel the same or worse after three or four days, it may be time to see your doctor.

This was mentioned before, but on account of importance, allow me to repeat myself. The body moves, exists, builds, repairs, maintains itself, and relies on the quality of the building material that we feed it to do just that. These fuels are vitamins. The right place to find vitamins is, of course, in the food that we eat. Unfortunately for many reasons, not all food is up to scratch nutrition wise on account of the type of soil, for instance, neglected soil deprived of nutrition as well as myriad other reasons. Another factor is we do not eat all the different foods that will provide the required variety of nutrients.

Imbalances occur, and for that reason a whole lot can go wrong with the body, from headaches to pain in your toe, to depression on account of a lack of some or other chemical in the brain. It can happen anywhere in the body. If you are not on a good quality multivitamin, now may be the time to do so; it may just be all that was needed in the first place. It stands to reason, if you have been taking vitamins or the recommended remedies and the problem persists, then it is time to see your doctor. Allow me to mention again that some vitamins may take a while to solve a problem. They work differently to allopathic medicines which are drug related and can be equated with shock treatment. The vitamins taken will not have been wasted, they will still provide you with a well-balanced metabolism.

A good multivitamin, including minerals, for the body as a whole, plus extra vitamin C, 300 mg, vitamin E, 400 i.u, (meant primarily for the vascular system, essential for red meat eaters). It may be possible to find a vitamin that includes that amount C and E, which is unlikely but not impossible, is highly recommended. The extra vitamins are available separately. This is very important for optimum health. The quantities of nutrition that the body needs are minute compared to the amount of food we eat; it is the variety and quality that matters. Just spare a thought for the many different organs, muscles, bones, the endocrine system, the list is enormous, that all need their own combination of nutrition, which they rely upon as their food supply. They consume food just like we do, and if they are neglected they suffer malnutrition, just as we do should we not be fed adequately. Please note, I do not advocate the taking of large amounts of vitamins supplements. That should come from the food we eat.

The suggestions on health and well-being offered here are few if one considers attacks by the hordes of ailments that can befall a person. Albeit the trut,h this is not a medical journal and was not the main purpose of this writing. That will require many volumes, which are available, and should one become interested in the different subjects regarding health, I can wholeheartedly recommend such action. It will not be regretted, and it will be a great deal of fun.

The purpose is merely to foster an interest and better understanding of the enormous role vitamins (nutrition) play in the workings and maintenance of the body, and to gain a better understanding of how the metabolism works. Hopefully, a better and healthier lifestyle with all the wonderful rewards and benefits will be the outcome.

To think that one will never again need assistance from a personal physician is also wishful thinking and a ludicrous idea. Doctors are and will always be our best friends. I am convinced they will wholeheartedly agree with all that is written in this book. This is why they are physicians, to help wherever they can, to prevent or relieve suffering, and provide what is only the best for everybody. That is the art of their nature.

There is a vitamin range that has proved itself an excellent product. It has been on the market for decades and has over the last ten years made astonishing progress. The product is of top quality and the range is enormous. It is such an outstanding product and the range so wide I am sure any health store owner or assistant will know what I am talking about.

Allow me to mention an instance where natural healing played an enormous role in my life due to an oversight. I suffered from burning eyes for a very long time. Several visits to eye specialists offered no comfort. The condition was extremely uncomfortable and painful. At long last the thought that my metabolism may be too acidic crossed my mind. What a light bulb moment, I thought of good old Celery seeds. A quarter teaspoon seed in a half glass hot water, left to cool and taken at bedtime. It did not take long for my eyes to be back to normal.

The final conclusion: Enjoy yourself, have fun, while at the same time derive enormous benefits from a moderate input from your side. This in the best economy of scale you will ever be offered, with unmatched benefits.

HOT AND COLD THERAPY

Another old favorite I have used for many years, and I don't think I will exaggerate if I say a ninety-five percent success rate, can be applied to a wide range of discomforts, mainly muscle or joint injuries and tired eyes (not recommended for open wound injuries) .

My greatest success with this treatment is with any kind of headache. The treatment is as follows. Have a jug of very cold water containing lots of ice ready, stand in the shower if available, otherwise use a basin. Allow water as hot as you can tolerate without scalding yourself to run over your head until you feel you have had enough. Turn off the hot water and immediately but slowly pour the ice cold water over your head. Once should be enough. Not only does it relieve headaches, it is terrific for refreshing the whole mind and body after a tiring spell at work or play.

For a twisted ankle: prepare a bucket of cold water with a lot of ice (very cold), a second bucket of hot water, as hot as you can tolerate. Put the injured ankle into the bucket and leave it there until you no longer feel the heat. Transfer the ankle to the other bucket full of ice cold water and leave it there till you no longer feel the heat. Repeat three or four times every three to four hours. One can suffer a wide range of ankle injuries. It is, however, possible that it is simply too badly damaged and professional help would be the only way out. You have tried, it may just have been sufficient.

TIRED EYES

Wrap a block of ice in a thin wet cloth and hold it against the eyes. Move it around and a lovely refreshing sensation will soon replace the tired feeling. Another way would be to fill a small plastic bag with water and leave it permanently in the refrigerator. Hold it against the eyes and cool comfort will soon be felt. If a small bag is not available, fashion one from the corner of a larger bag, tie the top together with a rubber band or string.

RESTORED VITALITY

Feel refreshed super-fast. Take a really hot shower, turn off the hot water, then turn on the cold water immediately at full force. The first time round it may be the worst physical shock you have ever experienced. Persevere, allow cold water to flow over your body, however not too much. Don't allow the core temperature of your body to be affected. The tingling feeling afterward is exhilarating and you will feel like a new person.

How does this remedy work? Increased vitality is created by the stimulating effect the fluctuating temperature has on the cells and tissue, as well as the increased blood circulation. Blood flow in one direction only, from the heart through the arteries, and to the heart through the veins. The hot water leaves the area depleted of blood, so after the cold therapy has been applied, the area that is now below body temperature needs to be warmed up. Fresh blood flows back to the blood depleted area to bring the temperature back to normal. Blood is loaded with nutrients and healing takes place rapidly and the tissue is stimulated by the changes in temperature. When something is stimulated, a new surge of energy is released and everything functions so much better.

REFLEXOLOGY

A form of therapy I also found fascinating when I first came across it many years ago. Reading and becoming familiar with the chapter on nerves will be of benefit to understand how this therapy works

Once more it demonstrates how important the nerve system is in the overall functioning of the body.

Sometimes, like a computer the organs and connecting nerves becomes a little log-jammed, and need to be rebooted or reprogrammed. It is extremely interesting how this works. Every organ in the body is connected via the nerves to a spot at the bottom of the feet. By massaging these spots, the functions of the organs are reprogrammed and restored, and at the same time causes the organs to shed any toxins that may be present and so restores them to perfect working condition. By simply walking or being active is nature's way of keeping the organs happy and in good working order, a major reason to keep active so keep walking. It is impossible to overwork the body, it will have exactly the opposite reaction. As previously emphasized it will become stronger.

For the same reason, it is advisable to walk barefoot as often as possible. It is exactly what I do, the moment I set foot inside my front door my shoes come off,

There are sandals or shoes available with pimples on the inside of the soles and are known as reflexology or health shoes.

Another way to stimulate the nerves when and where necessary is to massage that particular nerve, for instance, to relieve the pain in a sore muscle. Find the sore spot, usually where the nerve runs over a bone in shallow tissue, and massage it rather hard and vigorously.

This is painful, but persevere, it is usually not for very long and the pain will dissipate relatively quickly.

Headaches caused by eyes strain: Put the thumb and middle finger on either side of the head, find the hollow on the temple immediately behind the eyes. Squeeze as hard as you can possibly bear. Hold for as long as you can and relax. Repeat a few times.

Another treatment for the same problem: Push both thumbs right next to each other into the hollows above the eyes right next to the nose, as hard as possible. Repeat a few times.

SPORTSMEN and WOMEN

RAPID HEALING, INCREASED STAMINA, AND ENHANCED RESISTANCE TO INJURIES

Only the body can heal itself. No medical magic of any sort can recreate or make new cells to replace the dead or broken ones when injuries happen. Only the body can and that is the way healing takes place. Simple common sense.

Certain exercises or massaging and various other means of treatment can certainly speed up or enhance the healing process. Applying these actions promote blood flow. The blood is laden with nutrition. It goes without saying that the

more blood the injured area receives, the more nutrition, the faster will the injured area heal. Nature is indispensable during the healing process and nothing does the job better and faster when given the ideal conditions.

The strongest opposition to and what hampers the work the cells do and gets in the way of rapid healing, are of course toxins. On account of the fact they are both chemicals, the toxins which are really poison are very powerful, consequently forcing the cells to work harder to do the job of healing, and this requires more energy. Moral of the story: rid the body of all toxins.

Does it not stand to reason if there were no toxins in the vascular system, in other word, the entire body, the cells, tissues and consequently the organs, muscles, etc., would it not be so much stronger, and injuries would not occur that easily? And if they do occur, healing will be so much faster.

An equally important aspect to look at is stamina. The body is designed to operate at its best under certain conditions, and this must surely be when it is in a state of perfection; in other words, as pure and clean as possible, free of all toxins. It stands to reason that unencumbered cells free of toxins will be able to function and perform so much better. Who will reap the benefit? Fibres, tissues, muscles, organs, eventually the whole body of course.

Stinging nettle is ideal for detoxing. A suggestion would be to drink the whole, including the leaves, once or twice a month; even much more often if need be (completely harmless); one level teaspoon full finely crushed leaves in a glass of boiling hot water, left to cool and taken at bedtime.

I am well aware of the fact that contact sports require bulk and physical strength, hence the intake of vast amounts of meat being necessary. The fact that meat is highly toxic does not mean the problem is insurmountable. Herbal blood cleansers can be taken on a regular basis **plus the consumption of lots of fruit**. Fruit does the job superbly.

Although preferable, not for a moment do I advocate the elimination of meat in the diet, which is usually a hard act to follow. The reduction in the amount of meat consumed could be of benefit. To sustain the required amount of protein, I would suggest the introduction of vegetable protein, like soya or weigh (milk) protein.

Take care that it is pure protein, and not the additive enriched kind that can lead to situations where the sporting authorities would be in disagreement. Additive enriched protein is meant for body building.

The body uses the majority of its energy to digest food. Giving it something that is easier to digest than meat, could definitely be of benefit. Vegetable protein will most definitely require less energy to digest. *The most powerful animals are all vegetarians and the difference between human and animal DNA is only about 3%.*

Fruit contains a huge amount of sugar, or more to the point, fructose which is, of course, harmless sugar and is highly beneficial in as much as it is a perfect carbohydrate and supplies a sustainable energy release. *The increased stamina must be experienced to be believed.*

Chapter 22

SUMMARY

IS THIS REALLY TOO MUCH?

By now some folk may feel this much writing and what is recommended in this book is just too much of an effort and not worth their while. Not so. What is suggested here is something for everybody, from the person who simply wants to be healthy and full of energy without changing his/her lifestyle too much, to the person who wants to make a start at turning his/her life around and become serious at the art of good body and mind maintenance; or someone who would like to go the whole hog and reach their full potential as an athlete. From here you can move on to levels where professional advice or even coaching will be the next stop for you.

We all have to do is start somewhere. As for the folk who have been inactive with an "I don't really care" attitude towards life, hopefully your interest has been touched sufficiently enough to spur you on to action, no matter how small, and enjoy a more meaningful and more satisfied life from now on.

Whatever level you want to reach is entirely up to you. The book is aimed at making the whole range of society a more active and health-conscious and a very much healthier, happier and overall a more contented one. *One tends to aim for the moon, and if you hit the rooftops, you can consider yourself successful.*

This is a point where I have an opinion very different to almost every health adviser I ever heard of or met, (could the reason be financial?) and that is, I do NOT support the enormous emphasis placed on exercise to lose weight. Certainly, exercise is of the utmost importance to me as is evident throughout everything I have written. BUT that can wait, losing weight IS MUCH MORE IMPORTANT.

To lose excess weight (to put it bluntly, fat) via the exercise route, can only be lost by "melting" away the fat, and that will require enormous effort, more than you can muster at this stage. Be sensible and lose the excess weight first. Every kilogram in excess puts the heart under stress when the body is exercised. The worst the situation, the worst the potential damage to the heart. You are literally promoting heart problems.

When the excess weight has been shed, it is so much easier to exercise. I have often watched with intense interest how a personal instructor works day after day with a candidate to lose weight with minimal or no success. The end result? The candidate eventually becomes discouraged and comes to the conclusion: "It is expensive and it doesn't work for me," never to try again to lose weight.

It is very difficult to do exercises when one is overweight, and not the time to develop a love affair with any physical activity. Certainly not strenuous exercises, which I have no doubt the candidate will eventually reach if taken along a sensible and more comfortable route that will lead to the desired outcome. Once a person has developed a negative attitude towards anything, it can only be changed with an enormous amount of persuasion and hard work.

As little as just using an exercise bicycle in front of the television or whatever you choose to do is a good beginning. What I do emphasize to lose weight is primarily a healthy diet. Weave the fresh fruit and raw vegetable scenario in with your present diet and then slowly change for the better. Anything in the extreme is not necessary, move at your own pace. What usually happens is that such a person notices progress, feels so much better, observes the all-around improvement, then moves on to the next step. I am of the opinion that exercise is emphasized enough for the person to realize how important it is to achieve good health and happiness.

Whatever level you stay at, or move on to, is entirely up to you. Hopefully, I will have inspired or encouraged many people to reach for new heights by boosting their participation in sport, not merely for the love of sport and the benefits one will enjoy, but also a completely new lifestyle with new interests.

Keep to your regular diet if it is a reasonable one. If it is your choice, don't discard your love for meat. Just make a few sensible adjustments and add to it the suggestion of a lot more salads. A quick and easy one is the addition of a large glass of delicious vegetable or fruit smoothie, or a large cup of raw hot soup, once a day if possible. Why not eat all your fruit and vegetables in that manner? Include exercise, as little or as much as you like; the choice is yours.

On average, modern society is incredibly laid back and blasé about life. We cannot expect to **always take the easy way out** by doing the absolute minimum, or only eat what is "nice," in other words, food that has through bad eating habits becoming the preferred choice. Sometimes we have to make that little "sacrifice" to improve matters. The last suggestion is one such "sacrifice." This "sacrifice" always pays huge dividends, much more than the investment one makes.

Now for a very important misunderstood remark. Often, when the topic, detoxing, becomes relevant for discussion, the immediate reply I get without exception is, "I am very regular." This is not the point. There are two systems at work here. Being regular concerns the digestive system. Yes, that clears the body of waste and the kidneys and liver filters out the impurities. Unfortunately, the filtration system cannot cope on its own on account of the vast amount of unnatural and poor quality food we eat, and it still needs assistance, Refer to the chapter on Digestion where "a body clean on the inside" is mentioned.

Now the second system becomes relevant, the vascular system, which *means primarily cleaning and purifying the blood, removing all toxins to avoid the accumulation of all kinds of chemical build-up that can turn into many different negative conditions, which can take on many different characteristics all over the body. Could arthritis, among others, be one of them (just a thought)? How else can a body that has been designed not to get sick acquire this wide array of ill-effects the human race is afflicted with on a regular basis? The only way for these ingredients that create these adverse conditions in the body is through the mouth. Ever heard of "We dig our grave with our teeth"?*

In a "clean on the inside" body, in other words, the vascular system that covers every tiny nook and cranny, every cell, every muscle, every joint, when there is no poison anywhere in the system, then it stands to reason there is nothing to contaminate the blood and create problems. Would that perhaps prevent the dreadful conditions which may be painful, arthritis, and similar conditions, from forming? I would think so.

The blood reaches every single cell in the body and this is where the danger lurks; that is where you find the toxins and poisons that are so often referred to that create all the health problems that manifest themselves on the inside of the body. Cleaning the inside and keeping it clean, also known as detoxing, can be found in what is probably the most important chapter in the whole book, a chapter devoted entirely to this subject. Even if you understood it the first time round, read it again. That is the most important adjustment towards better health you will ever make in your lifetime.

Vegetarians need not be concerned, provided they eat a fair amount of raw fruit and vegetables, which is usually the case. For folk with a different outlook but still a little concerned about good health, I suggest a level teaspoon of dried crushed herbal leaves (Stinging nettle – if not available, ask for a substitute) taken as described before. It is not all that palatable, but what are a few seconds of unpleasantness when good health and lots of pleasure is at stake. The difference it can make to your overall health is enormous, not to mention feeling like a million dollars. **Repeat once a month**. A vast difference should soon be noticed.

This bit of advice can be noted by those who are really not into the health kick scenario and prefer a more sedentary lifestyle as their choice of an easier way to achieve improvement in their lives. At least you will be making an effort to keep your body cleaner on the inside than it probably ever has been. *Even that will be a gigantic move in the right direction, a host of benefits.* The energy your body needs to fight the odds against the unnatural negative conditions in your system is now available for use in a more positive way.

This is especially relevant to prospective mothers. Make sure your body is clean on the inside before, or as soon as possible after you become pregnant. Give your child the benefit of the maximum quality of your reproductive system you can possibly manage, the better the condition of your reproductive system the better chances are of producing a healthy happy baby.

Even if you are already on the way to becoming a mother, it is not too late, you can still do something worthwhile towards a positive result.

Good nutrition is the golden rule, and this cannot be stressed enough. It is of universal importance, more so at the time when we reach old age and hang on to every bit of good health we can muster. When organs are looked after the way they should be, life can be so much better. Think of the eyes and the brain as examples; you can see better, you can think more clearly than the average person your age. *It is not possible for organs that are so delicate to perform optimally when contaminated with toxins*. Surely just these two examples, among a multitude of others, should be enough to make one want to live life with a more responsible attitude.

Nothing can come into existence, develop, and grow without being fed to maintain good health. Even pot plants need food to flourish; deny them food and they will soon become yellow and wilt. They may not die, but are certainly not very happy campers. Feed them, and you have a display of beauty. This is a law that applies universally to every living entity.

Toxins, like any other impurities, are usually forced into and accumulate in between the tiniest of crevices, for instance where bones meet or are very close together. If left undisturbed long enough, they become compacted and eventually form crystals, and can very well turn into problematic conditions; for instance, what may be arthritis. Where the blood is clean, this is not possible.

By denying toxins the chance to exist in the body, you deny many problems the opportunity to establish a foothold.

Now I have said all I wish to say, there is one final comment I would like to make, and that is at the age of seventy-six, I have no idea what it is to be tired. This morning I walked a distance of plus minus ten kilometers at a brisk pace. After lunch, I did not feel like being idle, looked for something to occupy my time and decided to wash my car and clean it thoroughly inside and outside. Life is truly wonderful when at this stage one can still feel like a healthy and fit (not average) thirty-year-old, although taking care of one's well-being should start as early in life as possible, improvement can and will be noticed no matter what age you currently are.

There, but for the grace of God go I; very true, that adds to the obligation <u>we</u> have to do <u>our share</u> in creating the conditions and opportunities that will make it possible for us to enjoy the best life has to offer.

Be grateful and give thanks for what you have received free, gratis, and for nothing from our heavenly Father. It is incumbent upon us to at least respect and look after our bodies adequately.

Just as a matter of interest my personal statistics are: Age, 76, 1.82 m tall 90 k g B/P 120/75 H/r 50 beats per minute. Please don't see this as boasting, it is simply to show what is possible with a little dedication and discipline. This can be for everybody; well, let's say for the vast majority.

You can perform a mini E.C.G. on yourself. The pulse rate is the perfect tool to gauge your level of fitness and health in general, and by taking it daily(before a meal) you will become aware of any discrepancy immediately; for instance, a missed beat, not necessary an indication that all is not well. Should that be noticed several times per minute, then it is best you see your physician.

That is the first assessment a doctor makes, For instance, if your pulse rate rises above the regular by five to ten beats per minute, no need to be alarmed; it is an indication that things could be better or it may be due to a stressful situation. Should you feel a little jittery as well, it may be your heart has to work that little bit harder. It is an indication that your blood is a little lean. A spoonful of molasses for a day or two should bring the viscosity back up to normal, an easy and safe way to self-diagnose. Should the symptoms disappear and normality has returned, no extra measures are needed.

If your pulse rate is normally substantially higher and any of the above discrepancies appear, it would be advisable to see a doctor.

Thanks to the grace of a great and glorious God, the past twenty years have been the most wonderful of my entire life. My mind, which I consider my most valuable possession, has provided me with some of the most enjoyable moments; its fruitfulness, enlightened feeling, and clarity have sometimes astonished even me. What can I put it down to? My own opinion and conclusion would be that I practice what I preach.

Should you be fortunate enough to have a near perfect body, give thanks to the Lord for such blessings by doing your best to look after i. Remember, you are more than likely responsible for any breakdown of that incredible creation by not respecting it enough and having taken it for granted, in many instances for a very a very long time. Treat it with a little more respect and it may well surprise you with a lot of unexpected blessings.

Finally, what would be your ultimate measure of success? Very simple, when you spend no more than ten minutes on the toilet every day or at most every second day, you can claim success. Your system is operating at optimum efficiency level. When your mind feels as though it is open at the top and exposed to the universe and you are experiencing an energy level completely alien to most retired folk, you have arrived. Ccongratulations' (This condition is the ultimate of achievements; do not develop a sense of guilt if it is less than 100% percent of what you 7expected) simply work at it.

On average, at birth metabolisms are all the same and react in the same way, but due to difference in lifestyle, the whole body including chemical reactions, will be different from person to person. Should you have any doubt about partaking in any part of the program consult with your physician first. It is recommended you experiment with small quantities first, including exercises.

Allow me to mention that all the recommendations as far as the taking of herbal or any other products including vitamins, as well as exercises, are totally and completely innocuous. Nevertheless, you partake in all that is recommended and suggested entirely at your own risk. I do absolve myself of all blame whatsoever of any adverse consequences you the reader may suffer when partaking in any of the suggested programs.

ENJOY A QUALITY LIFESTYLE TO CREATE MEMORIES TO FEED OFF DURING OLD AGE.

About the Author

Steven Watson lives in Durban, South Africa, and lives for the outdoors. The principles in this book are part of his lifestyle and he still leads an active outdoor lifestyle at the age of 76. He feels like a healthy 30-year-old and believes rejuvenation is possible for **everybody** at any age.

www.ingramcontent.com/pod-product-compliance
Lightning Source LLC
Chambersburg PA
CBHW060246290526
45789CB00001B/214